Physical Fitness and Nutrition during Growth

....
Medicine and Sport Science
Vol. 43

Series Editors   *J. Borms*, Brussels
                  M. Hebbelinck, Brussels
                  R.J. Sheppard, Toronto, Ont.

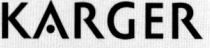

Basel · Freiburg · Paris · London · New York ·
New Delhi · Bangkok · Singapore · Tokyo · Sydney

Physical Fitness and Nutrition during Growth

Studies in Children and Youth in Different Environments

Volume Editors *J. Pařízková*, Prague
　　　　　　　 A.P. Hills, Brisbane

35 figures and 46 tables, 1998

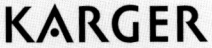

Basel · Freiburg · Paris · London · New York ·
New Delhi · Bangkok · Singapore · Tokyo · Sydney

Medicine and Sport Science

Published on behalf of the International Council of Sport Science and Physical Education
Founder and Editor from 1969 to 1984: E. Jokl †, Lexington, Ky.

Jana Pařízková
Laboratory of Health Promotion
3rd Clinic of Internal Medicine
1st Medical School
Charles University
U Nemocnice 2
CZ-12806 Prague (Czech Republic)

Andrew P. Hills
School of Human Movement Studies
Queensland University of Technology
Kelvin Grove Campus
Victoria Park Road
Kelvin Grove 4059
Brisbane, QLD (Australia)

Library of Congress Cataloging-in-Publication Data
Physical fitness and nutrition during growth: studies in children and youth in different environments /
volume editors, J. Pařízková, A.P. Hills.
(Medicine and sport science; vol. 43)
Includes bibliographical references and index.
1. Physical fitness for children – Cross-cultural studies. 2. Physical fitness for youth – Cross-cultural studies.
I. Pařízková, Jana. II. Hills, Andrew P. III. Series.
RJ133.P54 1998   613.7'042   dc21
ISBN 3-8055-6679-4 (hardcover: alk. paper)

Bibliographic Indices. This publication is listed in bibliographic services, including Current Contents® and Index Medicus.

Drug Dosage. The authors and the publisher have exerted every effort to ensure that drug selection and dosage set forth in this text are in accord with current recommendations and practice at the time of publication. However, in view of ongoing research, changes in government regulations, and the constant flow of information relating to drug therapy and drug reactions, the reader is urged to check the package insert for each drug for any change in indications and dosage and for added warnings and precautions. This is particularly important when the recommended agent is a new and/or infrequently employed drug.

All rights reserved. No part of this publication may be translated into other languages, reproduced or utilized in any form or by any means electronic or mechanical, including photocopying, recording, microcopying, or by any information storage and retrieval system, without permission in writing from the publisher.

© Copyright 1998 by S. Karger AG, P.O. Box, CH–4009 Basel (Switzerland)
Printed in Switzerland on acid-free paper by Reinhardt Druck, Basel
ISBN 3-8055-6679-4

Contents

VII **Preface**

1 **Growth, Development and Sociocultural Characteristics of Brazilian Preschool Children**
Rocha Ferreira, M.B.; Rocha L.L. (Campinas)

13 **Overnutrition, Undernutrition and the Body Mass Index: Implications for Strength and Motor Fitness**
Malina, R.M.; Katzmarzyk, P.T.; Siegel, S.R. (East Lansing, Mich.)

27 **Physical Fitness of 7- to 14-Year-Old Schoolchildren in Merida (Mexico) and Łódź (Poland)**
Siniarska, A. (Yucatan).; Jeziorek, A.; Nowakowska, M. (Łódź)

44 **Body Composition, Body Satisfaction, Eating and Exercise Behavior of Australian Adolescents**
Hills, A.P.; Byrne, N.M. (Brisbane)

54 **Sex Differences in Physical Fitness in Flemish Youth**
Lefevre, J.; Beunen, G. (Leuven); Borms, J.(Brussels); Vrijens, J. (Gent)

68 **Relationships between Physical Activity, Motor Ability, and Anthropometric Variables in 6-Year-old Estonian Children**
Oja, L.; Jürimäe T. (Tartu)

79 **Aerobic and Anaerobic Performances in Relation to Marginal Malnutrition and Altitude in Bolivian Boys and Girls**
Fellmann., N.; Bedu, M.; Coudert, J. (Clermont-Ferrand)

94 **Nutritional Status, Physical Fitness and Physical Activity in Children and Youth in Maputo (Mozambique)**
Prista, A. (Maputo)

105 **Evaluation of Physical Status of Children Living in the Zones of Influence of Small Doses of Radiation after the Chernobyl Accident**
Kozlova, K. (Vinnitsa)

117 **Growth and Motor Performances of Rural Senegalese Children**
Benefice, E. (Montpellier)

132 **Cardiorespiratory Fitness and Body Composition in Indian Children of 10–16 Years**
Khanna, G.L.; Majumdar, P.; Saha, M.; Mandal, M. (Bangalore)

145 **Treatment and Prevention of Obesity by Exercise in Czech Children**
Pařízková, J. (Prague)

155 **Methodological Considerations in the Assessment of Physical Activity and Nutritional Status of Children and Youth**
Hills, A.P.; Byrne, N.M. (Brisbane); Pařízková, J. (Prague)

161 **Conclusions and Perspectives**
Hills, A.P. (Brisbane); Pařízková, J. (Prague)

163 **Subject Index**

Preface

Concern for the development of the next generation has been a central theme in all civilizations, even the most primitive. Optimal health and a high level of fitness have long been recognized as the key to the future of any human population. Appropriate education, health care and stimulation during childhood are elements that encourage desirable morphologic, functional, metabolic and nutritional development of children. Specifically, a proper diet and an adequate level of physical activity for all individuals are essential factors for the achievement of this aim.

Unfortunately, there are substantial extremes identifiable in many parts of the world. Poverty and malnutrition are rife in countries of the Third World, whilst affluence in other areas, predominantly the industrially developed countries, has also provided enormous challenges. In the latter category, abundance and poverty often coexist. Similarly, the provision of a favorable environment with an ample diet, adequate education and health care is no guarantee that appropriate levels of physical fitness in children will be achieved. For example, there is an increasing prevalence of overweight and obesity in many countries.

The effect of malnutrition depends primarily on the degree, that is whether it is mild, moderate or severe, as reflected in times of famine or war. The onset and duration of malnutrition, as well as the degree and character, are also important factors in terms of an effect on physical performance. Components of fitness can be influenced in different ways. For example, marginal malnutrition causing smaller body size and greater leanness does not result in a marked deterioration of cardiorespiratory fitness but can have a more pronounced effect on muscular strength as this is dependent on muscle mass. Reductions in muscular strength may have an impact on economic productivity in the short and longer term. Notwithstanding the potential problems, there are also numerous examples of minimal or no ill effects in adulthood following marginal or modest malnutrition during the formative years.

Generally, the more pronounced the malnutrition, the more severe the consequences. At certain critical periods, for example during pregnancy and at times of weaning, the effect of deprivation can be more serious than at other periods of growth and development.

A reduction in spontaneous physical activity is generally the first line of defense in times of reduced energy intake. This has potentially significant consequences for motor, functional and morphologic variables characterizing physical fitness. There may also be social, psychological and intellectual components due to a lack of social contact and stimulation. Again, longer-term disruption may potentiate long-lasting effects which cannot always be compensated by realimentation. The incorporation of suitable physical activity during realimentation may also benefit the nature of the catch-up in growth and fitness.

The effects of an abundant diet and hypoactivity are well known. Low activity levels in particular, in industrialized countries, have contributed to an increasing proportion of overweight and obese children and adolescents. This has also impacted on functional capacity, fitness and predisposition for cardiovascular and metabolic diseases later in life. Unfortunately, there is no consensus amongst the scientific community regarding optimal levels of diet and physical activity for growth and development. An appreciation of the interplay of genetic factors and the environment is central to this area.

Observations of somatic, functional, motor, metabolic and nutritional development in children and youth living under different environmental conditions, following different ways of life, provide a nice framework for the variability of nutritional and physical fitness. These issues have been addressed in two previous scientific meetings and in monographs that emanated from these meetings. The first symposium was held in Zagreb (1989) as part of the 11th International Congress of Anthropological and Ethnological Sciences, and an initial monograph, *Human Growth, Physical Fitness and Nutrition*, was an outstanding Karger title edited by Shephard and Parizkova (1991). Proceedings of the second symposium, at the 13th International Congress of Anthropological and Ethnological Sciences in Mexico (1993) were published by the Institute Danone in Paris (1994). A wide cross section of authors from Algeria, Argentina, Brazil, Canada, China, Colombia, Cuba, Czechoslovakia, Hungary, India, Italy, Mexico, Poland, Senegal, Slovenia, South Africa, The Netherlands, Turkey and the USA contributed to these earlier volumes. This work has provided both an important insight into particular problems and some suggestions for improvement.

This third volume provides some new aspects and challenges for the optimal growth and development of children and youth of future generations all around the world. Contributions once again reflect the key status of children and youth in a diversity of challenging environmental contexts.

Jana Pařízková, Prague
Andrew Hills, Brisbane

Growth, Development and Sociocultural Characteristics of Brazilian Preschool Children

Maria Beatriz Rocha Ferreira, Lydia Luciana Rocha

Faculdade de Educação Física da UNICAMP – Cidade Universitária Zeferino Vaz, Campinas, Brazil

Introduction

The population variation and differential responses to environmental conditions are a challenge to the understanding of human adaptation. As the human species shows a remarkable range of plasticity in response to environmental stress and culture, the study of physical growth and development is a fascinating task.

Life in Latin America is difficult for a large proportion of the population. Malnutrition, infectious diseases, health care and unemployment are the main issues in these countries. Protein energy malnutrition (PEM), for instance, is an important factor affecting the physical growth and performance of children. At the consequential level, PEM might mean severe health impairment which is occasionally irreversible. PEM also has mild-to-moderate effects on health, especially when the stress occurs during the early years of life. These effects, however, are more difficult to quantify compared to the clinical manifestation of the severe forms. However, research has indicated that mild-to-moderate PEM in children is associated with infectious diseases, stunted growth, delayed maturation, reduced muscle mass, decreased working capacity, low levels of physical performance in tests of speed, strength, long distance runs, and throwing [1–9].

In Brazil there is a large difference between developed and underdeveloped areas, a factor which affects public services such as health care, education and sanitation, plus food availability. Whilst there is variation in the socioeconomic status of the population, the state of São Paulo is one of the more affluent areas in Brazil. Physical education is not part of the public preschool curriculum and is limited to children attending private preschools.

The main focus of public preschool programs is to develop fine motor performance to prepare children to write and read. Children spend a lot of time indoors, with few opportunities to play and to participate in physical activity outside. Similarly after school, the children have few opportunities for exercising at public facilities. This is in sharp contrast to the opportunities afforded upper class children whose parents may be able to afford membership of private clubs.

The purpose of this research is to study the growth, motor performance, psychological development, foodways and daily physical activity in 5- to 7-year-old Brazilian preschoolers of low socioeconomic status, living in São José dos Campos.

Methods and Subjects

Three hundred and ninety-one girls and 360 boys attending three part-time public preschools in São José dos Campos in the State of São Paulo, Brazil were studied. The growth and motor performance was measured during the period 1988–1994 (except in 1990). Surveys to determine sociocultural characteristics of children's families were administered in 1988, 1989, 1992 (only the food intake) and 1993. Psychological tests were completed in 1988, 1989, 1992, 1994.

Surveys were administered in the presence of each child's responsible adult using an adaptation of Rocha Ferreira protocol [9]. Information was gathered on food intake at home and school, food habits, economic status, illness, health treatment and motor activity. The recall method was used to estimate food intake over a 24-hour period [9]. In addition to the survey, a focus group was performed with a number of mothers to collect information on food habits, health and motor activity of children.

The graphic test of perceptual organization used was based on Bender's work. Bender proposed patterns of geometrical figures as a means of studying the visual motor skill of children. Nine geometrical patterns were originally presented from which Santucci [10] proposed five to be applied (the reader is referred to the description by Rocha Ferreira [9]).

Body image has been studied as an expression of human emotions. Goodenough [11] devised a test in which children were asked to draw a man from memory. The figure of a man was chosen because of its familiarity to children, and because male clothing is more uniform than that of women or children. This test does not require the use of language. As a child ages, his/her concept of the world develops accordingly and is reflected in more complex drawings. The evaluation is based on a quantitative analysis of proportions and spatial relationships of the position of the parts of the drawing with reference to each other and the total number of points awarded is translated into a scale [also see 9].

Growth status was analyzed using the anthropometric dimensions of weight, height, circumferences (arm and calf), skinfold thickness (biceps, triceps, subscapular, suprailiac, abdominal and medial calf) and breadths (bicondylar, biepicondylar, bicristal and biacromial). All measurements were completed on the left side of the body. Physical performance tests included standing broad jump, shuttle run, 20-meter dash and 30-second sit-up test reported elsewhere [9].

Results

Survey

There was little variation in food habits, daily physical activity and health problems of families comprising the study group. Whilst most families were intact with both mother and father, the mothers assumed a more important role in the household. Less than 10% of children lived only with the mother.

All families studied were from a low socioeconomic background but there was variation in the reported family income. The minimum monthly salary ranged from US$ 60 to 100, not enough for many to rent a house, buy food, clothes and medicine. Therefore, at least 50% of the families studied could be classified in the very low income category. The majority of families had 2 children, others 3 and 4 children.

Formal education of parents was also variable with 50% of the parents reporting completion of at least 1 of the first 5 years at school, which means that the majority could read and write. Most families claimed to own or be purchasing the predominantly two bedroom homes in which they lived. Residences were not slums and the water supply, garbage collection and electricity was under the aegis of public companies.

With regard to food habits, most children reported eating everything that was offered, although there was a variation in the quantity of food. In general, the mothers were responsible for the purchase of food and predominantly from the same supermarket in the neighborhood. Apparently budget restrictions prevented many from spending money on vegetables and fruits, therefore the open market (feira) was less frequented.

The 'merenda escolar', a state-wide meal program, was served daily, based on 300 kcal and 8 g of protein per meal for part-time school attendance. The children presented a large variation of estimated protein and energy intake at home (table 1). Boys tended to have higher estimated protein and energy intake than girls. Both sexes have estimated energy intakes below the recommendation and protein intakes that met the safe level according to WHO/FAO [12] and the Prague program [13]. Given the limitations of the 24-hour recall method, these results for estimated protein intake must be viewed with caution.

Children did not participate in any form of organized exercise program but completed a sound educational program at school focusing mainly on fine motor development. Daily physical activity comprised of playing in the home

Table 1. Mean values and standard deviations of estimated energy and protein intakes in preschoolers

	Energy, kcal		Protein, g	
	SJC	Prague	SJC	Prague
Girls				
Mean	1,840.5	2,182	77.6	71
SD	683.2	585	30.3	19.6
n	178	15	178	15
Boys				
Mean	1,961.7	2,194	85.4	74
SD	712.7	568	31.2	20.7
n	148	31	148	31

Recommended allowances for preschool children in Prague: 1,700 kcal and 65 g of protein. SJC = São José dos Campos.

environment, in the street or at friends' homes. More active games were pursued by boys and the majority of children reported a total of 1–3 h per day of television viewing.

Parents perceived their children to be healthy. Generally, only common ailments were reported. Accordingly, the majority of children did not present with any health problem that contraindicated participation in activity.

Psychological Development, Growth and Motor Performance

Most children displayed normal psychological development including maturity in body image and motor perception tests (table 2). A greater proportion of boys showed immaturity in both classifications.

Sexual dimorphism, whilst minimal at this age, exists. Boys tended to have slightly higher values for overall body size, sitting height, circumferences and breadths, lower values for skinfold thickness and performed slightly better on the physical performance tasks than girls (table 3).

Correlations of weight and stature with motor performance are presented in table 4. Correlations ranged from low to moderate in relation to stature with associations being significant for both sexes. After controlling for age and stature, the relationship between motor performance and body weight was low and negative for girls except for significant positive correlations for grip strength. Results were similar for boys.

Table 2. Frequencies and percentages of motor perception and body image tests in preschoolers from São José dos Campos

Classification	Scale	Girls		Boys	
		motor perception	body image	motor perception	body image
Significantly immature	1	20 (9.7)	16 (7.8)	24 (11.9)	24 (12.0)
Immature	2	38 (18.4)	47 (22.8)	32 (15.9)	60 (30.0)
	3	111 (53.6)	120 (58.3)	98 (48.8)	94 (47.0)
Normal	4	21 (10.1)	13 (6.3)	18 (9.0)	10 (5.0)
	5	17 (8.2)	10 (4.9)	29 (14.4)	12 (6.0)
Total	–	207 (100.0)	206 (100.0)	210 (100.0)	200 (100.0)

Figures in parentheses represent percentage.

The second-order partial correlations between stature and motor performance, after controlling for age and weight, are low to moderate, and they indicate that stature has a significant positive effect on motor performance, particularly in girls.

Zero order correlations among performance and psychological tests range from low to moderate, and the majority are significant (table 5). The shuttle run test presents the highest correlation with the other motor performance tests, followed by grip strength. The body image and visual perception correlation scores are low, but significant with shuttle run and strength test.

Discussion

The economic status of the group was variable but within the low socioeconomic class. The characteristic features of family behavior and associated problems are very similar to the population living in the capital [9] and in Ilhabela, an ocean island in the State of Sao Paulo [14].

The central role of the mother in household activities is consistent across studies conducted by the authors. There is some evidence of assistance on the part of a limited number of fathers. Estimates of food intake are similar to previous studies in the region [9, 14, 15] and suggest that on average, children may be energy-deficient. Unfortunately, the shortcomings of the 24-hour food

Table 3. Mean, standard deviations, number and t tests of anthropometric and performance characteristics of children from São José dos Campos and Prague

Variables	Age years	São José dos Campos						Prague			
		girls			boys			girls		boys	
		mean	SD	n	mean	SD	n	mean	SD	mean	SD
Age, years	4	4.6	0.20	13	4.7	0.20	18				
	5	5.5	0.30	109	5.6	0.20	98				
	6	6.6	0.30	199	6.5	0.30	189				
	7	7.2	0.20	70	7.2	0.20	55				
Weight, kg	4	18.4	3.10	12	18.7	1.40	18	18.3	3.47	19.2	2.86
	5	19.7	3.10	107	19.8	3.10	94	19.7	2.52	20.9	2.76
	6	21.0	3.00	193	21.2	2.70	186	21.6	2.81	22.1	2.68
	7	22.9	4.00	69	23.1	3.40	51				
Stature, cm	4	108.9	5.90	11	111.3	4.80	16	107.7	5.90	109.0	3.90
	5	113.4	5.80	109	113.6	5.10	95	112.8	4.40	113.5	5.80
	6	117.3	5.40	193	117.8*	5.20	183	118.6	4.90	119.2	4.10
	7	120.9	5.70	67	121.3	4.80	53				
Sitting height, cm	4	61.5	2.70	12	61.0	3.20	16	60.0	2.40	62.0	2.30
	5	62.8	3.70	109	62.6	3.20	95	62.5	2.50	63.8	2.70
	6	63.9	3.00	192	64.5*	3.10	184	64.7	2.80	65.5	2.60
	7	65.1	2.90	68	66.2	3.00	53				
Circumferences, cm											
Arm	4	16.3	1.10	12	16.6	0.80	17	16.9	1.40	17.2	1.20
	5	16.7	1.30	103	16.7	1.50	94	17.4	1.20	17.5	1.20
	6	17.0	1.30	195	16.9	1.30	183	17.7	1.20	17.7	1.10
	7	17.7	1.60	68	17.6	1.60	55				
Calf	4	22.3	1.20	12	22.4	0.90	17	22.9	2.20	23.4	1.20
	5	23.0	1.60	103	22.7	1.90	94	23.0	1.20	23.7	1.60
	6	23.7	1.80	194	23.6	1.80	182	24.5	1.60	24.1	1.10
	7	24.5	2.00	65	24.4	1.90	54				
Breadths, cm											
Bicondylar	4	4.3	0.30	11	4.5**	0.30	18	4.4	0.30	4.7	0.30
	5	4.5	0.30	102	4.7**	0.40	96	4.5	0.20	4.8	0.20
	6	4.6	0.30	195	4.7**	0.30	185	4.6	0.20	4.8	0.30
	7	4.7	0.30	69	4.9	0.30	55				
Biepicondylar	4	6.6	0.40	12	7.1**	0.40	18	6.9	0.40	7.3	0.40
	5	6.8	0.40	103	7.2**	0.40	95	7.0	0.30	7.4	0.30
	6	7.0	0.40	196	7.3**	0.40	185	6.9	0.50	7.5	0.30
	7	7.2	0.40	69	7.5**	0.40	55				
Bicristal	4	17.5	2.80	7	17.6	1.60	16	17.7	1.10	18.0	1.20
	5	17.3	1.10	73	17.7*	1.30	70	18.0	1.50	18.6	0.90
	6	17.9	1.10	144	18.1	1.00	122	19.2	1.10	19.4	0.90
	7	18.6	1.40	42	18.4	1.10	35				

Table 3 (continued)

Variables	Age years	São José dos Campos						Prague			
		girls			boys			girls		boys	
		mean	SD	n	mean	SD	n	mean	SD	mean	SD
Biacromial	4	24.3	2.10	7	25.1	1.90	17	24.3	1.40	24.6	1.00
	5	24.8	1.60	73	25.1	1.60	73	25.5	0.90	25.6	1.40
	6	25.7	1.60	141	26.0	1.60	122	26.1	1.10	26.2	1.00
	7	26.4	1.60	42	26.6	1.40	34				
Skinfold, mm											
Triceps	4	7.8	2.20	12	7.7	1.50	17	10.1	2.40	9.2	1.90
	5	8.5	2.20	103	7.7**	2.10	94	8.8	2.10	8.9	1.90
	6	8.5	2.20	194	7.3**	2.10	183	9.4	2.00	7.2	1.70
	7	8.9	2.40	68	8.1	2.90	55				
Subscapular	4	5.4	1.10	12	5.0	0.60	17	5.2	1.10	4.6	0.60
	5	5.5	1.40	103	5.3*	2.40	94	4.8	0.80	4.8	1.60
	6	5.8	1.70	104	5.0**	1.40	183	5.6	2.30	4.0	0.40
	7	6.3	3.00	68	5.5*	1.90	55				
Suprailiac	4	4.3	1.30	12	3.9	0.70	17	4.7	1.70	3.6	1.20
	5	4.6	1.50	103	4.1	2.80	94	3.5	0.90	4.0	1.70
	6	4.8	2.00	193	3.9**	1.50	183	4.9	3.20	3.0	0.60
	7	5.4	3.20	67	4.4**	2.00	55				
Calf	4	8.9	2.50	12	8.0	1.90	17	5.7	1.50	4.4	1.00
	5	9.8	2.30	104	8.6**	3.10	94	4.4	0.80	5.2	2.10
	6	9.7	2.60	194	8.2**	2.70	182	5.0	1.80	4.0	1.00
	7	10.7	3.50	67	9.0**	3.60	54				
Biceps	4	4.8	0.90	12	5.0	1.40	17	4.5	1.00	4.4	1.10
	5	5.7	1.60	103	5.0**	1.70	94	4.0	1.00	3.9	0.70
	6	5.8	1.80	194	4.9**	1.70	183	4.2	1.20	2.9	0.60
	7	5.8	1.80	68	5.2	2.10	55				
Sum	4	31.1	6.80	12	29.1	8.10	18	30.3	6.70	26.6	4.40
	5	34.2	7.60	103	30.6**	10.50	94	25.7	5.00	26.6	7.00
	6	34.5	8.70	194	29.2**	8.10	183	29.1	9.60	20.9	3.70
	7	37.1	12.50	68	32.1*	11.50	55				
Performance											
Jump, cm	4	82.6	14.30	10	81.9	20.00	12	71.6	15.70	75.5	12.80
	5	82.2	17.30	91	86.9	18.10	84	90.9	17.70	95.9	14.40
	6	93.9	18.70	183	100.7*	18.50	166	96.2	16.50	103.5	18.70
	7	98.6	18.70	61	102.9	19.10	50				
20-meter dash, s	4	6.1	0.9	10	5.7	0.7	14	6.2	0.70	6.0	0.80
	5	6.0	0.7	96	5.8	0.8	87	5.1	0.20	5.1	0.20
	6	5.7	0.6	191	5.4**	0.6	170	5.1	0.30	4.9	0.20
	7	5.6	0.6	66	5.3**	0.4	51				
Shuttle run, s	4	18.0	1.9	10	16.8	2.2	14				
	5	17.1	1.5	94	16.2**	1.5	87				
	6	15.8	1.4	190	14.8**	1.4	168				
	7	15.3	2	66	14.5**	1.1	48				

Table 3 (continued)

Variables	Age years	São José dos Campos						Prague			
		girls			boys			girls		boys	
		mean	SD	n	mean	SD	n	mean	SD	mean	SD
Sit-up (30 s)	4	2.1	2.30	11	3.6	4.20	12				
	5	5.4	4.20	94	4.9	4.10	84				
	6	6.4	4.00	181	8.3	4.60	162				
	7	6.2	4.30	60	9.1*	4.30	48				
Right hand grip, kg	4	9.4	2.80	7	9.5	2.80	15	7.5	2.40	10.5	2.20
	5	10.4	2.20	86	10.9	2.20	72	9.6	2.40	12.0	2.50
	6	11.5	2.30	144	12.8**	2.60	124	11.3	2.20	13.7	2.20
	7	12.5	2.60	41	14.3**	2.40	34				
Left hand grip, kg	4	8.4	3.40	7	9.1	2.80	15	7.2	2.50	10.0	2.00
	5	9.7	2.10	86	10.1	2.40	72	9.6	2.40	11.6	2.70
	6	10.7	2.30	142	12.1**	2.50	124	10.7	1.90	13.0	2.60
	7	11.8	2.60	41	13.1*	2.80	34				

In the Prague study there were 28 4-year-old, 39 5-year-old and 25 6-year-old boys and 25 4-year-old, 34 5-year-old and 25 6-year-old girls. Student t test: *$p<0.05$; **$p<0.01$ vs. girls.

recall procedures mean that estimated protein and energy intakes in this study may be misleading. The wide variation in reported food consumption is suggestive of individual metabolic demand, hereditary factors and adaptive processes affecting both energy input and output [16]. Males tended to have a higher food consumption than females, and participated in more exercise [9, 13, 14, 16].

The daily motor activities of the children were restricted by economic difficulties, lack of public parks and no physical education classes at school. Similar patterns of daily physical activity are observed in children from São Paulo and Ilhabela [9, 14]. Boys tended to be taller and bigger than girls, whereas girls tended to be fatter (table 3).

Skinfold thickness is more easily affected by measurement variation, and therefore, comparisons among studies should be completed with caution. The skinfold thickness values found in the present study are consistent with other studies from low socioeconomic background [4, 9, 13–15]. Boys had smaller skinfolds than girls in all samples. The smaller skinfold thickness of lower socioeconomic status children suggests either a deficit of energy intake and/or greater energy expenditure. Ethnic background, however, may be a confounding factor, given ethnic variation in subcutaneous fat distribution in the Brazilian population.

Table 4. Zero order and second order correlations between body size and performance tests in the present study and schoolchildren from São Paulo [9]

Tests	Zero order correlation				Motor performance and weight controlling for age and stature		Motor performance and stature controlling for age and weight	
	height		weight					
	girls	boys	girls	boys	girls	boys	girls	boys
Rocha Ferreira (age: 8.5 years)								
Number	60	84	60	84	60	84	60	84
Jump	0.12	0.03	−0.09	−0.01	−0.22	−0.06	0.24*	0.07
50-meter dash	0.14	0.21	−0.03	0.12	−0.13	−0.07	0.18	0.14
Shuttle run	0.31*	0.20	0.13	0.09	−0.07	−0.12	0.28*	0.19*
Grip	0.52**	0.47**	0.31**	0.48**	−0.03	0.19*	0.42**	0.14
Present study (age: 4–7 years)								
Number	218	193	218	193				
Jump	0.30**	0.40**	0.10	0.30**	−0.10	−0.20*	0.30**	0.20*
20-meter speed	0.30*	0.20**	0.20	0.30**	−0.10	0.10	0.10	−0.10
Shuttle run	0.30*	0.40**	0.20	0.30**	−0.10	0.04	0.20*	0.10
Right hand grip	0.60**	0.60**	0.60**	0.60**	0.40**	0.40**	0.10	0.10
Left hand grip	0.50**	0.50**	0.50**	0.60**	0.30**	0.40**	0.20*	0.10
Sit-up	0.20*	0.30**	0.01	0.30**	−0.10	0.04	0.20*	0.10

Signs for dash and shuttle run were reversed. *p<0.05; **p<0.01.

Boys performed better in motor tests and lack of motor activities for girls can partially explain the poorer response in motor tests. The standing broad jump, 20-meter dash and shuttle run scores are similar to those found in different studies [14–16]. In general, children from Prague [13] have better performance than individuals from São José dos Campos (table 3), except in the standing broad jump.

Low-to-moderate correlations may suggest that motor performance is not highly dependent on body weight and stature [17]. There are other variables affecting body dimensions and motor performance. The low correlation and the differences in the direction can probably be explained by the different backgrounds of the children, previous physical activity, nutritional status, and stimulation at home.

To better explain the relationship between morphological aspects and performance, second order correlation, controlling for age and either stature

Table 5. Zero order correlations among performance and psychological tests

Boys (n=112) Girls (n=119)	jump	20-meter dash	shuttle run	sit-up	right hand grip	left hand grip	body image	perception
Jump	1	*0.5***	*0.4***	*0.2**	*0.4***	*0.3***	*0.1*	*0.02*
20-meter dash	0.3**	1	*−0.5***	*0.1*	*0.3***	*0.3***	*0.1*	*0.02*
Shuttle run	0.4**	−0.5**	1	*0.2**	*0.4***	*0.4***	*0.3**	*0.4***
Sit-up	0.3**	0.4**	0.4**	1	*0.3**	*0.2**	*0.03*	*0.2**
Right hand grip	0.4**	0.3**	0.5**	0.4**	1	*0.8***	*0.2**	*0.3**
Left hand grip	0.3**	0.3**	0.5**	0.4**	0.8**	1	*0.1*	*0.3**
Body image	0.01	0.1	0.3**	0.01	0.3**	0.3**	1	*0.7***
Perception	0.01	0.2	0.3**	0.2*	0.3**	0.3**	0.7**	1

Signs for dash and shuttle run were reversed. Italicized figures represent girls. *p<0.05; **p<0.01.

or weight were calculated. Girls with higher body weight tended to have lower motor performance scores except in the hand grip test. This is consistent with the observation that movements in which the body is projected (such as standing long jump and dashes) tend to have low negative correlation with body weight [9, 15, 18].

Stature, when age and weight are controlled, has a significant positive correlation with jumping, agility, sit-up, and speed. These findings are similar to other studies done in different geographic areas [7, 9, 15, 18]. Stature as a proxy of biological maturation gives the idea that the more mature children have a better motor performance.

In conclusion the physical growth, physical performance and psychological status and socioeconomic characteristics studied are consistent with the marginal economic status of the families studied. Results point to the need for activities to foster the development of fine and gross motor performance and body image throughout the school program.

Summary and Conclusions

Growth, motor performance, psychological development, food habits and daily physical activity level were studied in 391 girls and 360 boys attending three part-time public day-care centers in São José dos Campos, the State of São Paulo during the period from 1988 to 1990. The following variables were assessed: (1) weight, height, circumferential measures (arm and calf), skinfold thicknesses (biceps, triceps, subscapular, suprailiac, abdominal and medial calf) and breadth measures (wrist, bicondylar, biacromial and bicristal), (2) performance tests (standing broad jump, shuttle run, 20-meter dash, handgrip strength and 30-second sit-ups, (3) survey of food intake at home and at school, food habits, economic status, medical history and motor activity of children; Santucci's proposition [10] of graphic tests of perceptual organization and body image using Goodenough's test [11]. The results showed that there was a small variation in the family behavior as regards food habits, daily physical activity, and also as regards medical history. Mothers demonstrated a central role in the household as compared with fathers, but some of the fathers had started sharing the household tasks with the mother, besides helping with the financial budget. A larger variation in family income, parental education and estimated energy and protein intake was shown. The psychological development of children was normal, only a small ratio of children showed lower levels as regards body image and motor perception tests. Results on somatic and motor developent also corresponded to the results of other studies from low socioeconomic classes. As regards gender differences, boys tended to have slightly higher values for overall body size, sitting height, circumferential and breadth measures, lower values of skinfolds and higher level of motor performance. Body weight tended to have a low negative correlation with broad jump and running tests, provided the effect of age and stature was excluded. A low positive correlation of stature with motor performance was also shown, when the effect of age and weight was excluded. A small variation in food habits in the family, daily physical activity and health problems demonstrates homogeneity and regularity in social behavior, similar to other populations living by the sea and in the city of São Paulo from the same socioeconomic class. However, children varied considerably in the estimated protein and energy intake at home. Boys tended to have a higher estimated protein and energy intake than girls. Both genders had estimated energy intakes below the recommendations that meet the safe level, which suggests that this population may suffer from energy deficiencies. The perceptual motor organization and body image scores are within the usual range of an average population. The perception test scores were a little higher than the scores for body image. This indicates a need for stimulation of the fine and gross motor performance and body image at school.

Acknowledgment

The authors gratefully acknowledge the financial support of CNP, FAEP and FAPESP/Brazil.

References

1 Frisancho AR, Guire K, Babler W, Borkan G, Way A: Nutritional influence on childhood development and genetic control of adolescent growth of Quechuas and Mestizos from the Peruvian lowlands. Am J Phys Anthropol 1980;52:367–375.
2 Rocha Ferreira MB, Zucas SM: Estado nutricional e aptidão física em pré-escolares. SEED-MEC – Ministerio de Educação e Cultura. Fundação Nacional de Material Escolar Prêmio Liselott Diem, 1991.
3 Spurr GB: Nutritional status and physical work capacity. Yearb Phys Anthropol 1983;26:1–34.
4 Malina RM: Physical activity and motor development/performance in populations nutritionally at risk; in Pollitt E, Amante P (eds): Energy Intake and Activity. New York, Liss, 1984, pp 285–302.
5 Malina RM: Growth and physical performance of Latin American children and youth: Socioeconomic and nutritional contrasts. Coll Anthropol 1985;9:9–31.
6 Malina RM: Motor development and performance of children and youth in undernourished populations; in Katch FL (ed): Sport Health and Nutrition. Champaign, Human Kinetics, 1986; pp 213–226.
7 Malina RM, Buschang PH: Growth, strength and motor performance of Zapotec children, Oaxaca, Mexico. Hum Biol 1985;57:163–181.
8 Rocha Ferreira MB, Rocha LL: Growth, physical performance and psychological characteristics of disadvantaged Brazilian preschool children; in Duquet W, Day JP (eds): Kinanthropometry IV. London, Spon, 1993, pp 256–267.
9 Rocha Ferreira MB: Growth, Physical Performance and Psychological Characteristics of Eight Year Old Brazilian School Children from Low Socioeconomic Background; doctoral dissertation, University of Texas at Austin, 1987.
10 Santucci H: Prova gráfica de organização perceptiva para crianças de 4 a 6 anos; in: Zazzo R, et al. (eds): Manual para o exame psicológico de crianças. São Paulo, Mestre Jou, 1981, pp 396–439.
11 Goodenough FL: Testes de inteligência infantil por meio do desenho da figura humana. Buenos Aires, Paidos, 1957.
12 World Health Organization: Energy and protein requirements. Report of a Joint FAO/UNU Expert Consultation. Tech Rep Ser. Geneva, World Health Organization, 1985, No 724.
13 Pařízková J, Adamec A, Berdychová J: Growth, Fitness and Nutrition in Preschool Children. Prague, Charles University, 1984.
14 Rocha Ferreira MB, Eilert CA, Silva PTN, Tavares S, Matsudo VKR: Physical growth and performance: Motor activity and foodways in Brazilian preschool children. 4th World Academic Conference on Human Ecology, Merida, 1993.
15 Rocha Ferreira MB: Physical growth and performance: Physical activity and foodways in Brazilian preschool. Proceedings of the 14th Congresso Panamericano de Educação Física, Costa Rica. San Jose, Memoria Volumen, 1993, vol 1, pp 1:290–297.
16 Pařízková J: Human growth, physical fitness and nutrition under various environmental conditions; Shephard RJ, Pařízková J (eds): Human Growth, Physical Fitness and Nutrition. Med Sport Sci. Basel, Karger, 1991, vol 31, pp 3–19.
17 Malina RM: Anthropometric correlates of strength and motor performance. Exerc Sport Sci Rev 1975;3:249–274.
18 Rocha Ferreira MB, Malina RM, Rocha LL: Anthropometric, functional and psychological characteristics of eight-year old Brazilian children from low socioeconomic status; in Shephard RJ, Parizkova J (eds): Human Growth, Physical Fitness and Nutrition. Med Sport Sci. Basel, Karger, 1991, vol 31, pp 109–118.

Dr. Maria Beatriz Rocha Ferreira, Faculdade de Educação Física da UNICAMP –
Cidade Universitária Zeferino Vaz, CP 6134, Campinas, SP 13.081–970 (Brazil)

Overnutrition, Undernutrition and the Body Mass Index: Implications for Strength and Motor Fitness

Robert M. Malina, Peter T. Katzmarzyk, Shannon R. Siegel

Institute for the Study of Youth Sports, Michigan State University, East Lansing, Mich., USA

Introduction

Excessive fatness negatively impacts performance tasks in which the body is projected through space, as in the long jump, vertical jump, or dash, and in which the body must be supported or lifted in space as in the flexed arm hang-ups or pull-ups [1, 2]. Overweight and/or relatively fat children as a rule do not perform as well in such events. On the other hand, overweight children are absolutely stronger, reflecting their larger body size, including muscle mass [3, 4].

In contrast, reduced body mass is characteristic of children with chronic mild-to-moderate undernutrition, who also show absolutely lower levels of muscular strength and motor performance [5, 6]. The reduced body mass reflects both reduced muscle mass and fatness. Given the association between muscle mass and strength, power and speed, different relationships with performance items may be expected in children reared under conditions of chronic undernutrition [7–9]. Thus, relationships between body mass and strength and motor performance in some cases of both overnutrition and undernutrition may be altered.

Further, in the context of public health, there is considerable interest in identifying children and youth who are overweight or underweight, or are at risk of becoming so. Emphasis on overweight is more common in developed countries, given the increased prevalence in overweight and/or obesity in children and youth over the past 2 decades [10–12]. On the other hand, emphasis on underweight is more common in developing countries because it reflects to a large extent low muscle mass, the work-producing tissue of the body.

The body mass index (BMI) is widely used in population surveys as an indicator of fatness [13–15] as well as chronic undernutrition [16–18]. The BMI includes both lean and fat components, and has different significance under conditions of overnutrition and chronic undernutrition. Although the BMI is used regularly with adults in developed and developing countries, and with children and adolescents in developed countries, it has not been widely used with children in developing areas characterized by conditions of chronic mild-to-moderate undernutrition.

In the context of the preceding, relationships between the BMI and the strength and motor fitness in contrasting samples of children were compared: (1) American children 6–13 years of age with a history of good nutritional status, and (2) rural Mexican children 6–14 years of age with a history of chronic mild-to-moderate undernutrition. The BMI was also used as the criterion for overweight, normal weight and underweight for the purpose of comparing the strength and motor fitness of children so classified.

Materials and Methods

Sample

The BMI, strength and motor fitness of three samples of children were considered: 440 black children 6–13 years of age (African American ancestry, 215 boys, 225 girls), 375 white children 6–13 years of age (largely south and central European American ancestry, 204 boys, 171 girls), and 373 Mexican children 6–14 years of age (Zapotec ancestry, 181 boys, 192 girls).

The American children represented cross-sectional samples from a larger mixed-longitudinal sample studied in Philadelphia in 1965 and 1966 [19]. The original project was approved by the Philadelphia Centre for Research in Child Growth (now the Wilton M. Krogman Centre for Child Growth) of the University of Pennsylvania and school officials. Parental permission was also granted for each child to participate in the study. The white children were from an upper middle class background, while the black children were from a lower middle class background. However, mean stature and body mass of the black and white children approximate the 50th percentiles of US reference data for each age and sex.

The Mexican children represent most of the primary school children in a rural Zapotec-speaking community of approximately 1,700 inhabitants in the Valley of Oaxaca in southern Mexico. The growth and performance status of the children was surveyed in 1978 [20]. The study was approved by the Institutional Review Board of the University of Texas at Austin, and community and school officials in the field. All children attending school were invited to participate in the study. The nutritional status of the community is at best marginal. The State of Oaxaca in southern Mexico has a history of poor nutrition, including a high prevalence of third degree malnutrition (Gomez scale) and a low mean per capita intake of protein and calories in school children. Estimated protein and energy intakes in the community are lower than recommended levels for Mexico. The marginal nutritional status of the community is also reflected in (1) high crude death rates, (2) especially high infant mortality

(152/1,000 live births), and (3) small statures and body masses relative to reference data for the US (approximately 5th percentiles) and Mexico [21].

Measurements

Stature (cm) and body mass (kg) were measured, and the BMI (kg/m^2) was calculated. Chronological age was calculated from birth and observation dates. Left and right grip strength (three trials with each hand) were measured with a Narragansett dynamometer in the American black and white children and with an adjustable Stoelting dynamometer in Zapotec children. The best values for right and left grip were added to provide a composite measure of grip strength. Motor fitness was assessed with a 35-yard dash with a stationary start (speed and power, better of two trials was used) and a standing long jump (power, explosive strength, best of three trials was used).

Intraobserver technical errors of measurement for stature and body mass were 0.48 cm and 0.27 kg, respectively, in the American children [22]. Corresponding technical errors for stature and body mass in the Zapotec sample were 0.33 cm and 0.10 kg, respectively, while interobserver errors were 0.67 cm for stature and 0.20 kg for body mass [9, 20]. Within-day reliability coefficients of the strength and motor fitness items were calculated as the correlation between the best and second best trials within single year age groups by sex. Coefficients in American boys ranged from 0.79 to 0.98 for grip strength, 0.39 to 0.98 for the dash, and 0.72 to 0.95 for the jump. For girls, the values ranged from 0.79 to 0.97 for grip strength, 0.50 to 0.93 for the dash, and 0.79 to 0.96 for the jump [23]. Corresponding coefficients ranged from 0.63 to 0.97 for grip strength, 0.52 to 0.86 for the dash, and 0.88 to 0.94 for the jump in Zapotec boys, and from 0.51 to 0.94 for grip strength, 0.71 to 0.89 for the dash, and 0.82 to 0.94 for the jump in Zapotec girls [20].

Definition of Overweight and Underweight

Individual children in each of the three samples were classified as overweight, normal weight and underweight on the basis of the BMI using US reference data [24]. Overweight was defined as a BMI $\geq$ 85th percentile, while underweight was defined as a BMI $\leq$ 15th percentile of the reference data. A BMI > 15th and < 85th percentiles was classified as normal weight. In the recommendations of Himes and Dietz [14], a BMI $\geq$ 85th percentile is indicative of the risk of overweight and a BMI $\geq$ 95th percentile is indicative of overweight. For the sake of simplicity, a BMI $\geq$ 85th percentile was used to indicate overweight in the present analysis.

Statistical Analyses

All variables followed a normal distribution except for the BMI, which was transformed using the natural logarithm (ln). Differences in body size, strength and motor fitness between boys and girls and among ethnic groups were determined using analysis of covariance (ANCOVA) with age as the covariate. The BMI, grip strength, the dash, and jump were adjusted for the effects of age within each sex by using the following regression: $Y = age + age^2 + age^3$. The standardized (z-transformed) residuals were retained for further analysis. Correlations between the age-adjusted z-scores for the BMI and the strength and motor variables were computed to examine relationships across the entire distribution of the BMI. Values for the dash were inverted because a lower performance time was a better performance. Differences in the prevalences in overweight and underweight by sex and ethnicity were tested with the χ^2 statistic.

To investigate the relationships between the BMI, strength and motor fitness in the three categories of the BMI, forward stepwise discriminant function analyses were performed to determine which strength and motor fitness items best discriminated between underweight, normal weight, and overweight children. The three independent variables (grip strength, jump, dash) were forced into the analysis in a stepwise manner, resulting in three steps. Additionally, a classification analysis was used to determine the percentage of cases correctly classified as underweight, normal weight or overweight based on the strength and motor fitness items.

Results

Growth status, strength and motor fitness of the children by sex within each ethnic group are summarized in table 1. There are no significant differences (ANCOVA with age as the covariate) in body size between boys and girls within each ethnic group, but boys have significantly better performances in grip strength, the dash and jump than girls in each ethnic group. Black and white children are, on average, significantly taller and heavier than Zapotec children within each sex ($p<0.05$). Black children are taller than white children within each sex ($p<0.05$), but body mass does not differ. Within each sex, the BMI, on average, does not differ between white and black children and between black and Zapotec children; however, the BMI of white children is significantly greater than of Zapotec children. It is clear that in absolute terms, Zapotec children are smaller than black and white children, but, on average, they have appropriate mass-for-stature as reflected in the BMI. Black and white children have significantly greater grip strength, run faster and jump farther than the Zapotec children; black children run faster than white children, and black boys perform better than white boys in the jump.

Results of the correlational analysis are summarized in table 2. Age-standardized z-scores for the BMI are positively and significantly ($p<0.05$) associated with grip strength within each sex and ethnic group. The correlations for the BMI and grip strength are reasonably similar between sexes in each ethnic group. Alternatively, correlations between the BMI and the jump and dash are not consistent by sex and ethnicity. The BMI is negatively associated ($p<0.05$) with performance in the jump in white boys and girls and in black girls, and with performances in the dash in white boys and black girls. The other associations are variable in magnitude and not significant in the other groups. It is of interest, however, that the BMI is positively related to performances in the jump and dash in Zapotec children.

Prevalences of underweight and overweight in the three samples of children are summarized in table 3. The prevalence of overweight ranges from 3.9 to 14.7% in boys and from 6.8 to 14.2% in girls, while the prevalence of under-

Table 1. Growth and performance characteristics of the subjects

Group	n	Age, years		Stature, cm		Mass, kg		BMI, kg/m^2		Grip, kg		Dash, s		Jump, m	
		mean	SD	mean	SD	mean	SD	mean	SD	mean	SD	mean	SD	mean	SD
White															
Boys	204	9.4	1.8	132.9	10.4	30.2	7.3	16.9	2.2	39.6	9.0	6.5	0.8	1.32	0.24
Girls	171	9.1	1.8	130.8	11.4	29.1	7.5	16.7	2.2	34.3	8.6*	6.9	0.9*	1.21	0.22*
Black															
Boys	215	9.5	2.2	134.6	12.7	30.2	8.9	16.3	2.2	40.4	11.8	6.0	0.7	1.48	0.30
Girls	225	9.7	1.9	136.9	13.1	32.2	10.4	16.7	2.8	36.9	11.2*	6.3	0.7*	1.30	0.26*
Zapotec															
Boys	181	9.8	2.3	123.4	11.3	25.3	6.1	16.4	1.3	27.1	9.3	7.0	0.7	1.14	0.23
Girls	192	8.9	2.3	119.4	12.2	23.5	6.8	16.1	1.6	21.8	9.0*	7.9	0.8*	0.94	0.17*

Differences between ethnic groups are discussed in the text. * $p<0.05$ vs. boys (ANCOVA with age as the covariate).

Table 2. Correlations between age-standardized z-scores for the BMI and strength and motor fitness

Group	Grip strength	Jump	Dash[1]
White			
Boys	0.30*	−0.33*	−0.23*
Girls	0.20*	−0.27*	0.03
Black			
Boys	0.49*	0.07	0.03
Girls	0.45*	−0.18*	−0.14*
Zapotec			
Boys	0.32*	0.14	0.15
Girls	0.27*	0.14	0.03

* $p < 0.05$.
[1] Signs for the dash were inverted because a lower time is a better performance.

Table 3. Prevalence of overweight and underweight by sex within each ethnic group

Group	n	Overweight		Underweight	
		n	%	n	%
White					
Boys	204	30	14.7	27	13.2
Girls	171	17	9.9	21	12.3
Black					
Boys	215	18	8.4	49	22.8
Girls	225	32	14.2	61	27.1
Zapotec					
Boys	181	7	3.9	21	11.6
Girls	192	13	6.8	25	13.0

Overweight: BMI ≥ 85th percentile;
underweight: BMI ≤ 15th percentile of US reference data.

Table 4. Results of forward stepwise discriminant function analyses for weight status (underweight, normal weight, overweight)

	n	Step 1	Step 2	Step 3	Wilks' lambda	p
White						
Boys	204	Jump (12.5)	Grip (12.7)	Dash (9.0)	0.78	<0.001
Girls	171	Jump (5.0)	Grip (6.1)	Dash (5.0)	0.84	0.001
Black						
Boys	215	Grip (24.1)	Dash (12.4)	Jump (8.3)	0.80	<0.001
Girls	225	Grip (20.1)	Jump (15.4)	Dash (11.0)	0.76	<0.001
Zapotec						
Boys	181	Grip (5.2)	Dash (3.1)	Jump (2.3)	0.92	0.03
Girls	192	Dash (3.7)	Grip (2.7)	Jump (2.0)	0.93	0.07

Each entry shows the variable entered and the F value to enter the analysis.

weight ranges from 11.6 to 22.8% in boys and 12.3 to 27.1% in girls. Prevalence rates do not differ by sex within each ethnic group (white, p=0.34; black, p=0.052; Zapotec, p=0.40). There is, however, variation in the prevalence of overweight by ethnic group within sex. White males have a significantly higher prevalence of overweight compared to black (p=0.047) and Zapotec (p<0.001) males. Black males have a significantly higher prevalence of underweight compared to white (p=0.011) and Zapotec (p=0.004) males. Black females also have a significantly higher prevalence of underweight than white (p<0.001) and Zapotec (p<0.001) females, as well as a significantly greater prevalence of overweight than Zapotec females (p=0.017). It is of interest that relative to US reference data for the BMI, the prevalence of underweight is highest in black children. As expected, the prevalence of overweight is lowest in Zapotec children within each sex.

Results of the forward stepwise discriminant function analyses for discriminating among underweight, normal weight, and overweight children by sex within each ethnic group using the strength and motor fitness tests are given in table 4. All discriminant functions are significant in white and black boys and girls, and only in Zapotec boys (p<0.05). In the white boys and girls, the jump entered first as the most important discriminator, while in black boys and girls, grip strength was the most important discriminator. Grip strength was also the most important discriminator in the Zapotec boys, while the dash was most important in Zapotec girls.

Table 5. Results of classification analysis for classifying underweight, normal weight, and overweight children using strength and motor fitness variables

Group	Percentage correctly classified			
	underweight	normal weight	overweight	total
White				
Boys	63.0	46.3	70.0	52.0
Girls	66.7	42.1	70.6	48.0
Black				
Boys	69.4	37.8	61.1	47.0
Girls	62.3	36.4	65.6	47.6
Zapotec				
Boys	66.7	32.6	71.4	38.5
Girls	61.1	34.8	80.0	40.5

The ability to classify individuals as underweight, normal weight or overweight based upon strength and motor fitness items from the discriminant function analyses was explored using classification analysis. The results indicate that based upon only three strength and motor fitness items, between 61 and 80% of children are correctly classified as overweight, and between 61 and 69% of children are correctly classified as underweight (table 5). The percentage of correct classifications for normal weight children is lower, ranging from 33 to 46%. The results thus suggest that the three strength and motor fitness items correctly classify children at the extremes of overweight and underweight. There do not appear to be ethnic or sex differences in correctly classifying children as underweight. However, fewer black children are correctly classified as overweight than are white and Zapotec children, and more Zapotec girls than boys are correctly classified as overweight based on strength and motor fitness items.

The standardized canonical coefficients derived from the discriminant function analyses are presented in figure 1. Note that the sign for the dash has been reversed since a lower time indicates a better performance. Grip strength loads positively on the discriminant function in every case, whereas the jump loads negatively in white children of both sexes, black girls, and Zapotec boys. The dash loads positively or negatively on the discriminant function with no apparent pattern. However, it should be noted that except for the low negative loading on the jump in Zapotec boys, all other canonical coefficients are positive in Zapotec children.

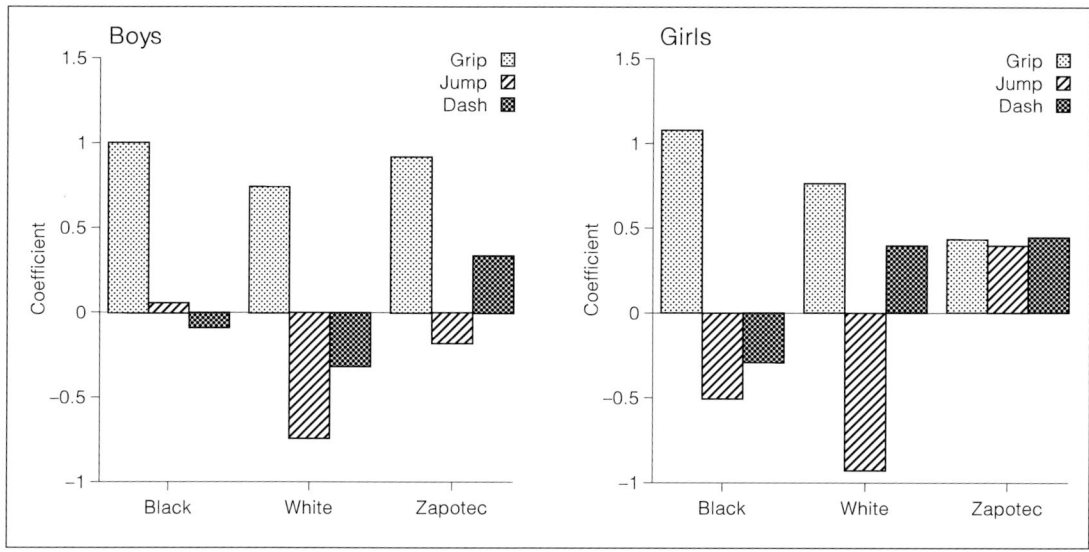

Fig. 1. Standardized canonical discriminant coefficients for the discrimination of weight status in boys and girls within each ethnic group from strength and motor fitness items.

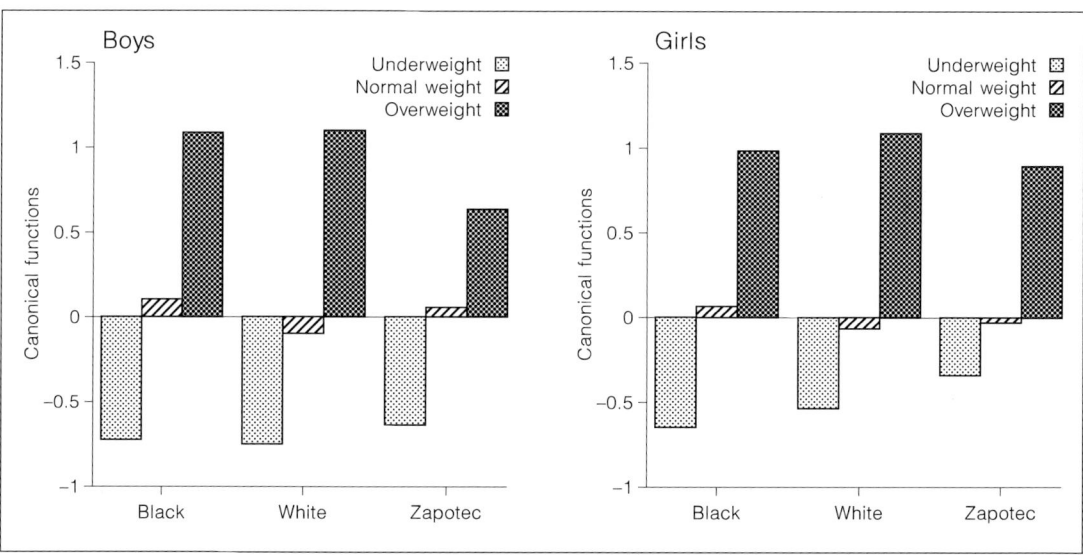

Fig. 2. Canonical functions evaluated at group centroids (means) for underweight, normal weight and overweight boys and girls within each ethnic group.

Figure 2 presents the canonical functions evaluated at the group centroids for underweight, normal weight, and overweight children. Within each ethnic group and in both boys and girls, the underweight group is characterized by negative functions, whereas the overweight group is characterized by positive functions. The normal weight group demonstrates functions which approximate zero. The results thus indicate a gradient from underweight to overweight for grip strength and motor fitness.

Discussion

The BMI is positively related to muscular strength in both sexes within each ethnic group. Correlations range from low (0.20) to moderate (0.49), emphasizing the role of body size in static strength in both well-nourished and mild-to-moderately undernourished children. Correlations for the standing long jump and 35-yard dash are more variable. Among the better nourished American white children, the BMI is negatively correlated with jumping performance in both sexes, and with the dash in boys. Among the better nourished American black children, the BMI is negatively related to jumping and running performance only in girls. Correlations for black boys approach zero. The results thus suggest that a larger BMI tends to have a negative influence on the performance of tasks requiring the projection of the body in well-nourished children. The lack of association between the BMI and jumping and running performance in black boys may be related to their lower BMI, on average (table 1), and lower prevalence of overweight (table 4) compared to white boys and black girls.

In contrast to the better nourished American children, correlations between the BMI and jumping and running performance, though low and not significant, are all positive in Zapotec children. The lack of a negative influence of the BMI on performances involving displacement of body mass in these mild-to-moderately undernourished children may be suggestive of a threshold level above which excessive fatness (i.e., a high BMI) exerts a negative influence on performance. The trends suggested by the correlations also highlight the important contribution of lean tissue to the BMI.

Observations of well-nourished young adult males indicate a curvilinear relationship between an index of physical fitness (based on scaled scores for seven items of strength and motor fitness) and the BMI [25]. The highest composite fitness score (372) was obtained by those with a BMI between 20.2 and 22.2 kg/m^2. Lower fitness scores were obtained by those with a low BMI (19.0–19.7 kg/m^2, 360) and with a high BMI (24.7–27.0 kg/m^2, 343). In the present analysis, the relationship between the BMI and strength and motor fitness was linear in boys and girls in each ethnic group. This may suggest that the association between the BMI and physical fitness varies with the age of the subjects. Unfortunately, corresponding data for young adult women are not available.

As indicated in the introduction, overweight during childhood and adolescence is routinely described as a major problem in developed countries and in some segments of developing countries (usually the upper socioeconomic classes). Similarly, underweight associated with chronic undernutrition is a major problem in developing countries. Using US reference data for the BMI, the prevalence of overweight ($\geq$85th percentile) and underweight ($\leq$15th percentile) was estimated in the three samples of children. Those with BMIs between the 15th and 18th percentiles were classified as normal weight.

The prevalence of overweight is generally low (table 3) compared to more recent samples of children and adolescents [26]. Note, however, that the sample of black and white children was surveyed in 1965–1966. More white boys than girls were classified as overweight, while more black girls than boys were classified as overweight. Further, among white girls, the underweight group was significantly older than the overweight group ($p < 0.05$). The observations for girls probably reflect the contrasting social class backgrounds of the samples, and are consistent with the inverse association between social class and overweight in girls and women which has been documented since the 1960s [27, 28]. A contributing factor may be early dieting and emphasis on weight control in well-off girls 10–13 years of age.

It is of interest that the sample of Zapotec children living under conditions of chronic mild-to-moderate undernutrition includes a small number of overweight children. In both the black and Zapotec children, the prevalence of overweight in girls is almost double that in boys, while the opposite is evident in the white children. At the other extreme of the BMI distribution, the prevalence of underweight is almost identical in white and Zapotec children, while black boys and girls have almost double the prevalence.

Among Zapotec children of both sexes, the underweight group was also significantly older than the overweight group ($p < 0.001$). This probably relates to the later maturation in the sample so that, relative to the reference data, the Zapotec children have less mass for stature in the early adolescent years. The adolescent spurt occurs first in stature and then in body mass so that there is a temporary period where body mass lags relative to stature.

There is considerable current interest in identifying children at risk of becoming overweight [14]. Overweight children were identified with 60–80% accuracy based on only three strength and motor fitness items in the present analysis. Perhaps better discrimination would be possible if more fitness items were used. Similarly, the limited battery of strength and motor fitness items also correctly classified about 65% of the underweight children.

The standardized canonical coefficients derived from the discriminant function analyses (fig. 1) and the canonical functions evaluated at the group centroids for underweight, normal weight and overweight (fig. 2), taken together, indicate a gradient from underweight to overweight such that grip strength increases and the standing long jump decreases, while trends for the dash are more variable. Thus, there are clear differences in strength and motor fitness between underweight, normal weight and overweight children. The results are consistent with other studies which indicate that overweight children are stronger than normal children due to their larger body size, and that excess fatness impacts negatively those events in which the body is propelled through space, in the jump [3, 4]. Note, however, that there is some variation in the discriminant function analyses among children in the three ethnic groups. Except for the low negative loading on the jump in Zapotec boys, all other canonical coefficients are positive in Zapotec children. This suggests that the BMI has a different meaning for the strength and motor fitness of the Zapotec children compared to better nourished American black and white children.

Although the Zapotec children are absolutely shorter and lighter than black and white children, their current weight for stature as reflected in the BMI is appropriate and compares favorably, on average, with those of the American children (table 1). This emphasizes the poor nutritional history of the Zapotec children, specifically in compromising their early growth. Most growth stunting associated with chronic undernutrition occurs in the first 2–3 years of life, and also includes reduced muscle and fat mass. This, of course, has implications for the interpretation of the BMI in developing countries, which has been highlighted previously for adults [16]. Similar cautions also apply to children. The BMI impacts the strength and motor fitness of adequately nourished children differently than it impacts corresponding measures in children with poor nutritional histories currently living under inadequate nutritional circumstances.

Summary and Conclusions

Relationships between the BMI and strength and motor fitness were compared in American children 6–13 years of age with a history of good nutritional status and in rural Mexican children 6–14 years of age with a history of chronic mild-to-moderate undernutrition. Age-standardized z-scores for the BMI are positively and significantly associated with grip strength within each sex and ethnic group. Correlations between the BMI and the jump and dash are not consistent by sex and ethnicity. The results suggest that a larger BMI tends to have a negative influence on the performance of tasks requiring the projection of the body in well-nourished children. The lack of a negative influence of the BMI on the performance involving displacement of body mass in the mild-to-moderately undernourished children may suggest a threshold level above which excessive fatness (i.e., a high BMI) exerts a negative influence on performance. The trend also highlights the important contribution of lean tissue to the BMI. The BMI was also used as the criterion for overweight, normal weight and underweight. There are clear differences in strength and motor fitness between underweight, normal weight and overweight children. Results of discriminant function analyses suggest that the BMI has a different meaning for the strength and motor fitness of the rural Mexican children compared to better nourished American children. The results also have implications for the interpretation of the BMI in developing countries, which has been highlighted previously in adults.

References

1 Malina RM: Anthropometric correlates of strength and motor performance. Exerc Sport Sci Rev 1975;3:249–274.
2 Malina RM: Anthropometry, strength and motor fitness; in Ulijaszek SJ, Mascie-Taylor CGN (eds): Anthropometry: The Individual and the Population. Cambridge, Cambridge University Press, 1994, pp 160–177.
3 Beunen G, Malina RM, Ostyn M, Renson R, Simons J, Van Gerven D: Fatness, growth and motor fitness of Belgian boys 12 through 20 years of age. Hum Biol 1983;55:599–613.
4 Malina RM, Beunen GP, Claessens AL, Lefevre J, van Eynde B, Renson R, Vanreusel B, Simons J: Fatness and physical fitness of girls 7 to 17 years. Obes Res 1995;3:221–232.
5 Malina RM: Physical activity and motor development/performance in populations nutritionally at risk; in Pollitt E, Amante P (eds): Energy Intake and Activity. New York, Liss, 1984, pp 437–451.
6 Malina RM: Motor development and performance of children and youth in undernourished populations; in Katch FI (ed): Sport, Health and Nutrition. Champaign, Human Kinetics, 1986, pp 213–226.
7 Malina RM, Little BB: Body composition, strength, and motor performance in undernourished boys; in Binkhorst RA, Kemper HCG, Saris WHM (eds): Children and Exercise. Champaign, Human Kinetics, 1985, vol 11, pp 293–300.
8 Malina RM, Little BB, Shoup RF, Buschang PH: Adaptive significance of small body size: Strength and motor performance of school children in Mexico and Papua New Guinea. Am J Phys Anthropol 1987;73:489–499.
9 Malina RM, Little BB, Buschang PH: Estimated body composition and strength of chronically mild-to-moderately undernourished rural boys in southern Mexico; in Shephard RJ, Parizkova J (eds): Human Growth, Physical Fitness and Nutrition. Basel, Karger, 1991, pp 119–132.
10 Troiano RP, Flegal KM, Kuczmarski RJ, Campbell SM, Johnson CL: Overweight prevalence and trends for children and adolescents. Arch Pediatr Adolesc Med 1995;149:1085–1091.
11 Freedman DS, Srinivasan SR, Valdez RA, Williamson DF, Berenson GS: Secular increases in relative weight and adiposity among children over two decades: The Bogalusa Heart Study. Pediatrics 1997;99:420–426.
12 Hughes JM, Li L, Chinn S, Rona RJ: Trends in growth in England and Scotland, 1972 to 1994. Arch Dis Child 1997;76:182–189.
13 Roche AF, Siervogel RM, Chumlea WC, Webb P: Grading body fatness from limited anthropometric data. Am J Clin Nutr 1981;34:2831–2838.

14 Himes JH, Dietz WH: Guidelines for overweight in adolescent preventive services: Recommendations from an expert committee. Am J Clin Nutr 1994;59:307–316.
15 Seidell JC: Obesity in Europe: Scaling an epidemic. Int J Obes 1995;19(suppl 3):S1-S4.
16 Norgan NG: Body mass index and body energy stores in developing countries. Eur J Clin Nutr 1990;44(suppl 1):79–84.
17 Ferro-Luzzi A, Sette S, Franklin M, James WPT: A simplified approach of assessing adult chronic energy deficiency. Eur J Clin Nutr 1992;46:173–186.
18 Immink MDC, Flores R, Diaz EO: Body mass index, body composition and the chronic energy deficiency classification of rural adult populations in Guatemala. Eur J Clin Nutr 1992;46:419–427.
19 Malina RM: Growth, Maturation and Performance of Philadelphia Negro and White Elementary School Children; doctoral dissertation, University of Pennsylvania, Philadelphia, 1968.
20 Malina RM, Buschang PH: Growth, strength and motor performance of Zapotec children, Oaxaca, Mexico. Hum Biol 1985;57:163–181.
21 Malina RM, Selby HA, Buschang PH, Aronson WL: Growth status of school children in a rural Zapotec community in the Valley of Oaxaca, Mexico, in 1968 and 1978. Ann Hum Biol 1980;7:367–374.
22 Malina RM, Moriyama M: Growth and motor performance of black and white children 6–10 years of age: A multivariate analysis. Am J Hum Biol 1991;3:599–611.
23 Malina RM, Mueller WH: Genetic and environmental influences on the strength and motor performance of Philadelphia school children. Hum Biol 1981;53:163–179.
24 Must A, Dallal GE, Dietz WH: Reference data for obesity: 85th and 95th percentiles of body mass index (wt/ht^2) and triceps skinfold thickness. Am J Clin Nutr 1991;53:839–846.
25 Welon Z, Jurynec R, Sliwa W: Ciezar nalezny mezczyzn. Mat Prace Antropol 1988;109:53–71.
26 Malina RM, Katzmarzyk PT: Validity of the body mass index as an indicator of the risk of overweight and of overweight in adolescents. Am J Clin Nutr, submitted.
27 Goldblatt PB, Moore RE, Stunkard AJ: Social factors in obesity. JAMA 1965;192:1039–1044.
28 Stunkard A, d'Aquili E, Fox S, Filion RDL: Influence of social class on obesity and thinness in children. JAMA 1972;221:579–584.

Robert M. Malina, Institute for the Study of Youth Sports, 213 IM Sports Circle,
Michigan State University, East Lansing, MI 48824–1049 (USA)
E-Mail RMALINA@PILOT.MSU.EDU

Physical Fitness of 7- to 14-Year-Old Schoolchildren in Merida (Mexico) and Łódź (Poland)

Anna Siniarska[a], Anna Jeziorek[b], Maria Nowakowska[b]

[a] Department of Human Ecology, CINVESTAV-Merida, Yucatan, Mexico and IE, PAN, Warsaw, Poland;
[b] Department of Physical Education and Health, Łódź University, Łódź, Poland

Introduction

Physical fitness is not necessarily positively correlated with body build. There are examples of boys living in poor socioeconomic conditions (in Tunis), possessing unsatisfactory somatic development but with superior results in physical and motor performance to counterparts living in better socioeconomic conditions [1]. This phenomenon indicates that somatic and motor development can be an expression of adaptation to local living conditions which include nutrition and physical activity. Nutrition and rearing style have also been emphasized as a main problem in cross-cultural studies on physical fitness [2]. Comparative studies between Tunisian (Sfax) and Polish (Wrocław and Kraków) children of 9–18 years of age revealed that the taller and heavier Polish children also have better results in physical fitness performance than Tunisian children [3, 4]. Clearly, the examples above indicate that comparative studies should not only pay attention to the character of the human settlement (the nature of the city, town, village) but also the socioeconomic class [5], education and socioprofessional status of parents, family size and school type [6].

The main aim of the present study is a comparison of physical performance of Mexican and Polish children living in city environments of similar size, where living conditions and nutritional habits are very distinct. Significant differences also exist in the school physical education programs.

Table 1. Three-factor analysis of variance of somatic and physical fitness variables of primary schoolchildren from Merida (Mexico) and Łódź (Poland)

Somatic measures and motor tasks	F1 age (F)	F2 sex (F)	F3 ethnic group (F)	2-way interactions (F)			3-way interactions (F)	R^2/R
				EG-sex	EG-age	sex-age	EG-sex-age	
Body height	370.78***	1.70	514.13***	0.22	2.95**	2.16*	0.86	0.76/0.87
Body weight	161.95***	3.33	44.95***	0.01	2.34*	1.40	0.75	0.54/0.73
Arm circumference	62.57***	1.44	6.36*	2.75	0.36	0.90	0.82	0.31/0.55
Grip strength	95.91***	25.82***	1.43	8.10**	6.88**	2.31*	3.07**	0.41/0.64
Shuttle run	47.75***	132.26***	66.43***	29.12***	5.04***	2.21*	0.98	0.34/0.59
Vertical jump index	19.53***	68.17***	8.06**	1.06	6.54***	1.69	0.29	0.17/0.41
Spine flexibility index	1.47	20.71***	150.33***	19.86***	3.75**	1.19	0.99	0.15/0.39
Reaction time	3.54**	1.78	43.50***	9.05**	3.24**	3.05**	1.13	0.08/0.28

*p<0.05; **p<0.01; ***p<0.001.
F1 = Factor 1 (ethnic group: Mexico, Poland); F2 = factor 2 (sex: boys, girls); F3 = factor 3 (age: eight age groups from 7 to 14 years); F = F value; EG = ethnic group.

Materials and Methods

The sample consisted of 552 Mexican and 496 Polish elementary schoolchildren, 7 through 14 years of age. The children represented a cross-sectional sample studied in 1996–1997. Mexican children came from Merida (Yucatan state) and were mostly of Maya origin. Polish children came from Łódź, a city with a substantial textile industry. Both samples of children were representative of lower social stratum families. Three anthropometric dimensions were measured for each child: weight, stature and arm circumference. Physical fitness variables included right grip strength measured with a dynamometer; spine flexibility measured by the Groshenkov-Wolański instrument [7] [the difference in length of the spine in centimeters (cervicale-lumbale, CLU) in an upright and flexed (hands touch the floor with knees straight, CLF) position]; reaction time (in scores) measured by the Quickstick scale; measures of motor performance: the three-cycle shuttle run (running in a figure-of-eight around two flags placed 5 m apart), and Sargent jump [the difference between the height in the upright position with an extended hand (UH) and maximal vertical jump (JH) in centimeters measured on a scale attached to the wall]. Two indices were calculated, a flexibility index: CLF–CLU/CLU · 100 and a Sargent jump index: JH – UH/UH · 100.

The following hypotheses were tested in the study: (1) ethnic group, sex and age are related more to anthropometric measures than to strength, flexibility, reaction time and motor performance measures (dash and vertical jump) and (2) physical fitness variables which show significant changes between age groups are more dependent on body build measures than more stable ones. Analysis of variance was used in relation to the first problem and regression analysis for the second.

Table 2. Body height (in cm) of schoolchildren from the cities of Merida in Mexico and Łódź in Poland

Age group years	Sex	Merida (Mexico)				Łódź (Poland)				t test Mexico/Poland
		mean	SD	n	t test, m/f	mean	SD	n	t test, m/f	
7	m	113.98	4.6	44	NS	124.06	6.8	27	NS	***
	f	113.88	5.8	45		122.96	7.3	13		***
8	m	118.66	6.4	32	NS	129.12	5.7	33	*	***
	f	119.19	6.4	32		126.49	5.0	35		***
9	m	125.14	6.4	33	NS	133.81	6.1	36	NS	***
	f	126.21	7.2	31		132.42	6.1	31		**
10	m	129.87	6.3	42	NS	139.09	7.1	33	NS	***
	f	131.96	7.0	51		140.23	6.9	26		***
11	m	134.92	6.6	51	NS	141.94	7.5	51	*	***
	f	134.36	6.3	38		144.89	6.5	43		***
12	m	140.21	8.2	34	NS	150.60	7.6	42	NS	***
	f	141.17	7.5	34		151.94	7.4	39		***
13	m	142.28	9.6	33	NS	155.57	7.1	40	NS	***
	f	145.82	7.1	31		158.27	8.8	22		***
14	m	148.25	5.4	10	NS	163.65	7.6	13	NS	***
	f	144.07	8.4	11		159.04	4.3	12		***

*$p<0.05$; **$p<0.01$; ***$p<0.001$.
NS = Not significant; m = males; f = females.

Results

The proportion of total variation (R^2) of dependent variables is provided in table 1. Stature accounts for 76.6%, weight – 53.9%, grip strength – 40.9%, shuttle run – 34.5, arm circumference – 30.7%, Sargent vertical jump index – 17.2% and flexibility index – 15%. The smallest proportion is accounted for by reaction time – 7.7%.

There is a significant additive effect of both ethnic group and age on anthropometric measures (height, weight and arm circumference). For stature, the ethnic group factor has the strongest effect followed by age. There are two-way interaction effects between ethnic group and age, and sex and age (table 1). Table 2 indicates that taller girls and boys in each age group are seen in Łódź than in Merida. Age and ethnic factors have the strongest effect on weight and

Table 3. Body weight (in kg) of schoolchildren from the cities of Merida in Mexico and Łódź in Poland

Age group years	Sex	Merida (Mexico)				Łódź (Poland)				t test Mexico/Poland
		mean	SD	n	t test, m/f	mean	SD	n	t test, m/f	
7	m	21.75	3.0	44	NS	24.54	4.9	27	NS	**
	f	22.22	5.1	45		25.34	6.8	13		NS
8	m	23.38	3.9	32	NS	27.30	6.0	33	NS	**
	f	24.47	4.3	32		25.31	4.4	35		NS
9	m	26.73	5.0	33	NS	29.46	4.2	36	NS	*
	f	29.11	6.3	31		28.29	5.5	31		NS
10	m	30.57	5.4	42	NS	33.16	7.7	33	NS	NS
	f	31.77	7.6	51		33.86	6.8	26		NS
11	m	35.23	8.0	51	NS	36.05	8.0	51	NS	NS
	f	35.24	7.6	38		37.71	7.2	43		NS
12	m	38.45	6.9	34	NS	42.02	9.0	42	NS	NS
	f	38.18	7.3	34		41.84	9.7	39		NS
13	m	39.52	9.8	33	NS	44.98	9.1	40	*	*
	f	42.76	7.7	31		50.52	10.3	22		**
14	m	43.56	3.5	10	NS	49.78	8.8	13	NS	*
	f	42.69	7.9	11		50.36	7.1	12		*

*p<0.05; **p<0.01.
NS = Not significant.

arm circumference. There is only one significant interaction effect showing that ethnic group and age jointly affect the weight of the children studied (table 1). The differences in weight between Polish and Mexican children are not significant. Younger boys (7–9 years old) and children 13–14 years old are heavier in Łódź than in Merida (table 3). There is not a significant interaction effect of the three factors on arm circumference (table 1). Among 8- to 9-year-old boys arm circumference is significantly greater in Poland than in Mexico, and for the same age Mexican girls have greater arm circumference than boys (table 4). For grip strength, age followed by sex had the greatest effect (table 1) but there is a significant three-way interaction effect (ethnic group, age and sex factors). Among younger children, better results were found in Merida with significant differences between girls. In contrast, older boys from Łódź had significantly greater grip strength than boys from Merida (table 5). Sex

Table 4. Arm circumference (in cm) of schoolchildren from the cities of Merida in Mexico and Łódź in Poland

Age group years	Sex	Merida (Mexico)				Łódź (Poland)				t test Mexico/Poland
		mean	SD	n	t test, m/f	mean	SD	n	t test, m/f	
7	m	17.30	1.6	43	NS	18.15	2.2	27	NS	NS
	f	17.96	2.4	45		18.77	2.7	13		
8	m	17.70	1.6	32	*	18.76	2.2	33	NS	*
	f	18.65	1.9	32		18.41	1.7	35		
9	m	18.35	2.2	33	*	19.46	2.2	35	NS	*
	f	19.92	2.6	31		19.45	2.1	31		
10	m	19.73	1.9	42	NS	20.45	2.8	33	NS	NS
	f	20.28	2.7	50		20.37	2.4	26		
11	m	21.29	3.0	51	NS	21.29	2.7	54	NS	NS
	f	21.33	2.9	38		21.22	2.6	43		
12	m	21.81	2.2	34	NS	22.64	2.8	41	NS	NS
	f	21.61	3.7	34		21.69	2.6	39		
13	m	22.26	3.3	33	NS	22.49	2.8	40	NS	NS
	f	22.12	2.5	31		23.34	2.5	22		
14	m	22.22	0.8	10	NS	23.31	2.6	13	NS	NS
	f	22.68	3.0	11		22.79	2.4	12		

*p<0.05.
NS = Not significant.

differences are particularly marked in older Łódź children (from 11 years of age). Three factors have an additive effect on shuttle run. The sex factor represents the strongest effect and age the weakest. There are also three two-way interaction effects. Ethnic group with sex, ethnic group with age and sex with age jointly affect this dependent variable (table 1). Girls and older boys in Poland have faster (shorter) run times than children in Mexico. Sexual differences are marked (especially in Merida), with faster run times for boys (table 6). Three-factor analysis of variance in case of the Sargent jump index shows that there is a significant additive effect of three factors, sex showing the strongest effect followed by age and ethnic group. There is only one two-way interaction effect, ethnic group and age jointly affect this dependent variable (table 1). Whilst not statistically significant for all age groups, there is a tendency for the jumping performance in both sexes to be better in Merida children up to 9 years of age,

Table 5. Grip strength of right hand (in kg) of schoolchildren from the cities of Merida in Mexico and Łódź in Poland

Age group years	Sex	Merida (Mexico)				Łódź (Poland)				t test Mexico/Poland
		mean	SD	n	t test, m/f	mean	SD	n	t test, m/f	
7	m	8.23	4.4	35	NS	4.54	4.1	13	NS	NS
	f	7.26	2.4	31		2.88	1.2	8		***
8	m	8.92	3.4	26	NS	8.15	4.2	26	NS	NS
	f	8.44	3.5	27		6.00	4.0	28		*
9	m	12.36	4.5	33	**	8.52	4.1	33	NS	**
	f	9.00	3.6	29		9.43	9.4	28		NS
10	m	10.62	3.1	42	NS	11.69	4.1	32	NS	NS
	f	10.36	3.8	50		10.27	3.7	26		NS
11	m	11.86	4.5	51	NS	14.94	3.4	54	**	***
	f	13.03	5.6	37		12.77	4.0	43		NS
12	m	17.88	7.1	34	NS	19.19	5.0	42	***	NS
	f	15.85	6.0	34		15.05	4.4	39		NS
13	m	17.52	7.8	31	NS	21.85	6.2	40	*	*
	f	18.03	6.6	31		17.95	5.9	22		NS
14	m	16.80	8.0	10	NS	28.31	7.2	13	***	**
	f	15.64	5.3	11		17.50	6.0	12		NS

*p<0.05; **p<0.01; ***p<0.0001.
NS = Not significant.

and then the results in Łódź children are better. Better results were found in boys in most age groups, with statistically significant differences predominant in Merida (table 7). In the case of the spine flexibility index, there is an additive effect of two factors (ethnic group followed by sex) on this dependent index. There are also two, two-way interaction effects, ethnic group with sex, and ethnic group with age jointly affecting flexibility (table 1). Polish 7- to 9-year-old children display greater flexibility than Mexican children. The same is true for older girls. Sex differences are more marked in Mexico than in Poland (table 8). There is a significant additive effect of both ethnic group and age factors on reaction time, the ethnic group factor having the greatest effect. There are also three two-way interaction effects, ethnic group with sex, ethnic group with age and sex with age (table 1). Statistically significant differences are seen between girls in Merida and Łódź (table 9).

Table 6. Shuttle run (in min) of schoolchildren from the cities of Merida in Mexico and Łódź in Poland

Age group years	Sex	Merida (Mexico)				Łódź (Poland)				t test Mexico/Poland
		mean	SD	n	t test, m/f	mean	SD	n	t test, m/f	
7	m	19.38	2.2	44	*	17.85	2.0	26	NS	**
	f	20.79	3.2	44		18.18	2.1	13		**
8	m	17.13	2.3	32	NS	17.59	1.8	32	NS	NS
	f	19.53	3.5	32		18.10	1.6	35		*
9	m	16.59	1.8	33	*	16.70	1.4	35	NS	NS
	f	17.55	1.9	31		17.35	1.6	30		NS
10	m	15.88	1.5	42	***	15.89	1.2	33	**	NS
	f	17.35	1.5	51		16.77	1.3	26		***
11	m	16.41	1.6	51	**	15.96	1.3	52	NS	NS
	f	17.97	2.4	38		16.25	1.2	43		NS
12	m	15.67	1.2	34	***	15.43	1.5	39	**	NS
	f	18.85	2.9	33		16.42	1.3	39		***
13	m	15.52	1.4	33	***	14.91	0.8	40	*	*
	f	17.49	1.8	31		15.68	1.3	22		***
14	m	15.72	1.2	10	***	14.03	0.8	13	***	**
	f	18.76	1.7	11		15.38	0.7	12		***

*p<0.05; **p<0.01; ***p<0.001.
NS = Not significant.

The next step of the analysis relates to the influence of body build of children represented by stature, weight and arm circumference on physical fitness variables. The relationship between motor performance and anthropometry was evaluated by regression analysis of these three body measurements on each motor performance task. The coefficient of determination (R^2) was used to estimate the percentage of variance (PEV) of each motor performance explained by these three independent variables (fig. 1–4).

Generally it was found that body build parameters explain a greater PEV of physical fitness performance in Polish than Mexican children, and in girls rather than boys. Body build also shows a greater relationship with grip strength and shuttle run than with other physical fitness items. Among boys the PEV is the smallest at the age of 7 years in Merida and 8 years in Łódź and diminishes a little at the age of 13 years. The greatest PEV is observed

Table 7. Sargent vertical jump index of schoolchildren from the cities of Merida in Mexico and Łódź in Poland

Age group years	Sex	Merida (Mexico)				Łódź (Poland)				t test Mexico/Poland
		mean	SD	n	t test, m/f	mean	SD	n	t test, m/f	
7	m	12.89	3.4	43	NS	11.89	3.0	27	NS	NS
	f	12.46	2.9	44		11.33	4.2	13		NS
8	m	15.01	2.6	32	**	13.12	2.6	33	NS	**
	f	13.12	2.5	32		12.20	2.2	35		NS
9	m	15.35	3.2	33	**	15.00	2.4	35	*	NS
	f	13.33	2.5	31		13.50	2.7	31		NS
10	m	15.51	2.1	42	***	15.52	2.7	33	NS	NS
	f	13.53	2.3	51		14.33	3.7	26		NS
11	m	14.22	2.5	50	NS	15.54	2.5	52	NS	**
	f	13.19	2.9	38		14.73	2.8	43		*
12	m	15.67	3.3	34	NS	17.03	3.7	41	**	NS
	f	13.99	4.3	34		14.77	2.4	39		NS
13	m	15.73	3.2	33	**	17.15	3.1	40	NS	NS
	f	13.62	2.2	31		15.84	3.9	22		*
14	m	16.26	2.4	10	**	19.14	2.6	13	*	*
	f	12.70	2.7	11		16.33	2.5	12		**

*p<0.05; **p<0.01; ***p<0.001.
NS = Not significant.

at 14 years of age (fig. 1, 2). Among girls, the PEV tends to diminish at the age of 11 years (excluding grip strength in Poland and vertical jump in Mexico). Since the age of 12–13 years (earlier in Mexican girls) PEV of most motor performance tests increases, reaching the greatest values at the age of 14 years (fig. 3, 4).

Discussion

An understanding of the influence of the three factors, age, sex and ethnic group on body build and physical fitness variables depends on the definition of each factor. The factors studied do not have an independent impact on variables of body build and physical fitness but can be interrelated. The age

Table 8. Spine flexibility index of schoolchildren from the cities of Merida in Mexico and Łódź in Poland

Age group years	Sex	Merida (Mexico)				Łódź (Poland)				t test Mexico/Poland
		mean	SD	n	t test, m/f	mean	SD	n	t test, m/f	
7	m	19.28	8.6	44	NS	26.95	8.7	27	*	**
	f	17.27	8.6	45		32.25	4.1	13		***
8	m	20,47	10.6	32	*	28.75	9.2	33	NS	**
	f	14.61	8.0	32		29.59	8.9	35		***
9	m	19.89	8.9	33	NS	27.17	7.4	35	NS	***
	f	17.03	7.7	31		26.29	8.1	31		***
10	m	23.04	8.8	42	**	25.59	9.0	32	NS	NS
	f	17.99	7.9	51		24.18	7.8	26		**
11	m	21.01	9.4	51	*	23.93	9.1	54	NS	NS
	f	17.21	7.9	38		23.00	8.2	43		**
12	m	22.89	9.2	34	**	26.43	8.4	42	NS	NS
	f	17.08	6.6	34		22.88	7.9	22		**
13	m	24.71	13.4	33	*	26.04	9.1	39	NS	NS
	f	17.71	8.1	31		29.32	9.5	22		***
14	m	23.36	7.7	10	NS	25.15	8.8	13	NS	NS
	f	17.30	5.4	11		28.02	6.7	12		***

*$p<0.05$; **$p<0.01$; ***$p<0.001$.
NS = Not significant.

factor is mostly associated with developmental changes (ontogenesis) which are genetically controlled, but in very stressful conditions can be modified by environmental factors. The sex factor also has a biological basis, but its influence on physical fitness variables can also have a nonbiological basis (differences between sexes in physical activity, interactions between siblings, school and family mode of life) [8]. Ethnic group also has a genetic bias, but environmental conditions have a significant contribution. These conditions include differences in socioeconomic status (mostly in education and income), in way of life and nutrition, which partly depends on socioeconomic status but also on nutritional habits, so different in Poland and Mexico. The school physical education program is very different in both countries. Many poor Mexican children have permanent jobs in supermarkets during their 'free' time.

Table 9. Reaction time (in scores) of schoolchildren from the cities of Merida in Mexico and Łódź in Poland

Age group years	Sex	Merida (Mexico)				Łódź (Poland)				t test Mexico/Poland
		mean	SD	n	t test, m/f	mean	SD	n	t test, m/f	
8	m	8.59	1.0	13	NS	7.78	1.6	22	*	NS
	f	8.84	0.6	11		6.40	2.2	18		***
9	m	8.33	0.9	23	NS	7.97	1.4	33	*	NS
	f	8.44	0.9	18		7.09	1.9	31		**
10	m	7.91	1.2	39	**	7.75	1.0	29	NS	NS
	f	8.56	0.6	37		7.49	2.0	25		*
11	m	7.74	1.2	47	NS	7.32	1.1	53	NS	NS
	f	8.23	1.2	35		7.61	1.4	41		NS
12	m	7.32	1.1	33	NS	7.40	1.2	32	NS	NS
	f	7.90	1.4	34		7.81	0.9	39		NS
13	m	7.58	0.9	32	NS	7.12	0.9	39	NS	*
	f	7.80	1.3	29		7.05	0.7	22		*
14	m	7.65	1.2	10	NS	6.81	0.6	13	NS	NS
	f	7.92	1.0	11		6.97	1.0	12		*

*p<0.05; **p<0.01; ***p<0.001.
NS = Not significant.

The three-factor definitions in the case of physical fitness variables could be 'age', mostly a genetic factor, 'sex', a genetic and physical activity factor, and 'ethnic group', an environmental factor with some genetic bias.

Body build variables are very strongly affected by the age (genetic) factor. For weight and arm circumference this factor is in the first place followed by ethnic group. However, stature is more affected by ethnic group compared with age. This would suggest that any regulation of living conditions can very strongly affect stature, and also have an influence on weight and arm circumference. The sex factor does not play an important role in the case of body build variables in children 7 through 14 years of age.

Physical fitness variables are less sensitive to the three factors analyzed than height and body weight, as suggested in the first hypothesis. Age (genetic factor) followed by the sex factor mostly affects grip strength. The sex factor mostly affects shuttle run and vertical jump, whilst flexibility and reaction time are mostly affected by the ethnic group factor. These results suggest that

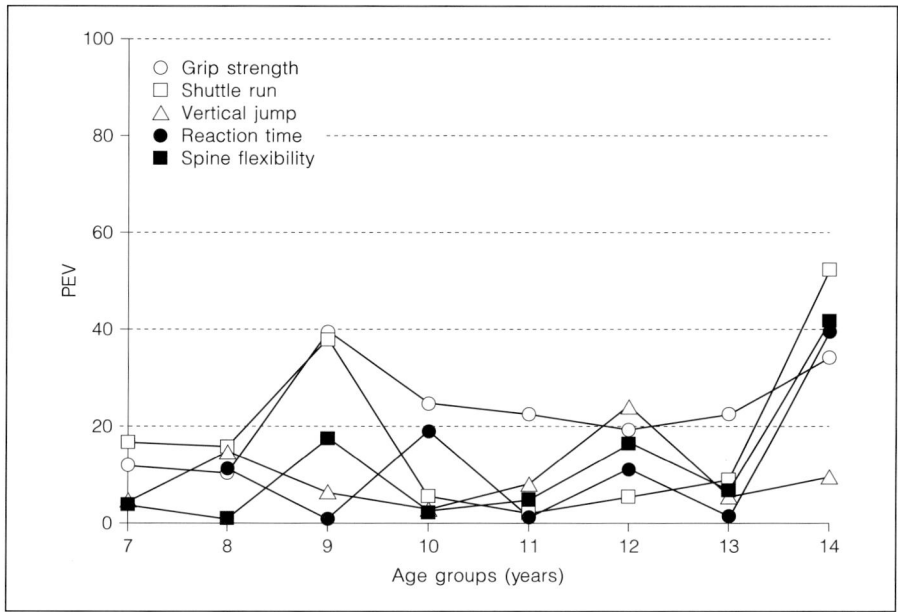

Fig. 1. PEV in physical fitness variables explained by the regression of the anthropometric measurements on each performance task (Mexican boys).

grip strength and shuttle run are probably more strongly genetically controlled than vertical jump, spine flexibility and reaction time, respectively. A high heritability of grip strength is also represented in the literature [8]. Studies based on similarities between siblings have revealed strong genetic links not only for grip strength and shuttle run, but also for flexibility and reaction time, and to a lesser extent for vertical jump [9]. In contrast, there are also findings that muscular strength and reaction time are rather weakly genetically controlled [10, 11]. This disparity underlines the difficulty of the biological and environmental determination of physical fitness and the variability in methodology to study these issues.

Grip strength and vertical jump results are superior in Mexican children at a younger age, and in Polish children at older ages. Both physical performance variables are weakly affected by the ethnic group factor, and there is a supposition that some genetic predisposition can influence this phenomenon. However, differences in the physical activity level between the two countries at various age periods cannot be excluded. Sex differences in these variables are also marked.

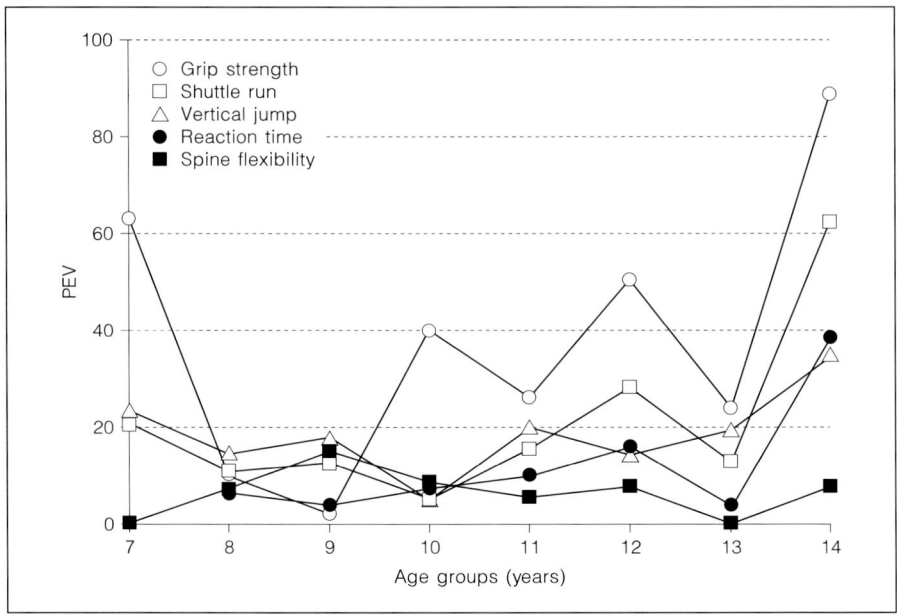

Fig. 2. PEV in physical fitness variables explained by the regression of the anthropometric measurements on each performance task (Polish boys).

For the shuttle run, spine flexibility and reaction time, the results achieved by Polish children (especially girls) are generally better than results achieved by Mexican children. These variables are affected by the ethnic group factor and the differences in living conditions might be largely responsible for these results. Sex differences in reaction time are not statistically significant, and there are no significant changes in spine flexibility with age. Flexibility of the spine shows a rapid development in very young children and changes very little during later ontogenetic development [9].

Comparative studies between Polish and Tunisian children have shown that somatic development in African children may be delayed by approximately 1 year. If a correction is made for this, differences in motor performance disappeared [3, 4]. Studies on girls' maturation have shown that in Merida the mean age of menarche is 12.09 years [12], whereas in Łódź the mean age is 13 years [13]. If a correction is made for differences in maturation (table 10) the results show even bigger differences in body build and physical fitness variables than differences observed for the same calendar age. Polish children are not only significantly taller but also heavier and Polish boys have significantly greater arm circumference. Results suggest that even when

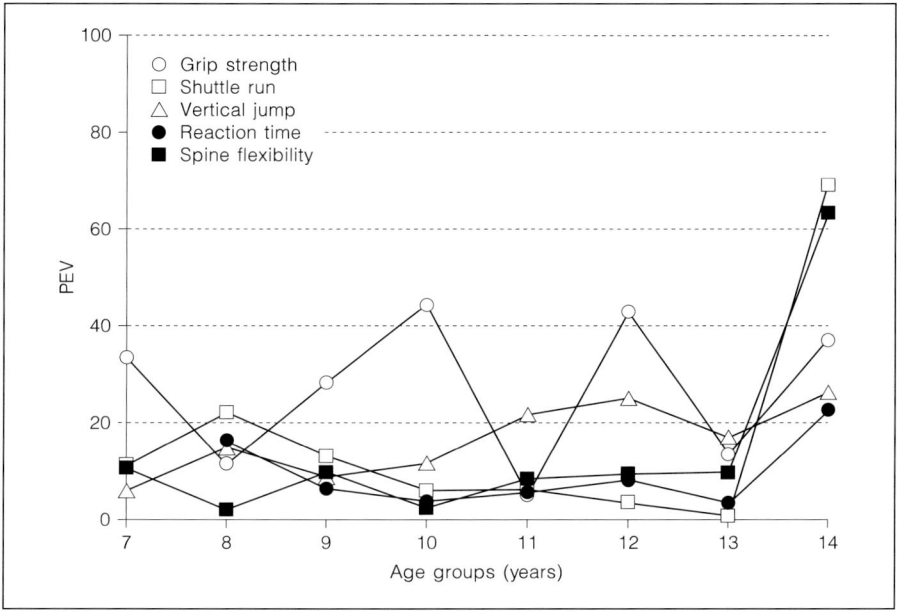

Fig. 3. PEV in physical fitness variables explained by the regression of the anthropometric measurements on each performance task (Mexican girls).

differences in biological development are eliminated, the observed differences in physical fitness results may depend on physical activity and environmental conditions such as life-style and nutrition.

As a general rule, if the influence of body build on motor and physical performance is greater, this indicates stronger genetic control [14, 15]. For almost all of the physical fitness variables studied, the PEV rises at the age of 14 years. It has been reported that the period of intense motor development is very sensitive to training [16]. It would also appear that during puberty, the intensive development of the organism might have an impact on motor performance, and that training may influence variables such as grip strength, running and jumping performance. The character and complexity of the performance tasks studied is also an important factor. Some motor and physical performance tasks also show significant changes with age. This includes grip strength (a static strength measure) which is associated with a small muscle group, the vertical jump (an example of explosive strength) which includes the work of several muscle groups, and shuttle run which depends not only on speed but also on the movement coordination respectively. Two other variables, spine flexibility and reaction time (more complex ones than the three above mentioned perfor-

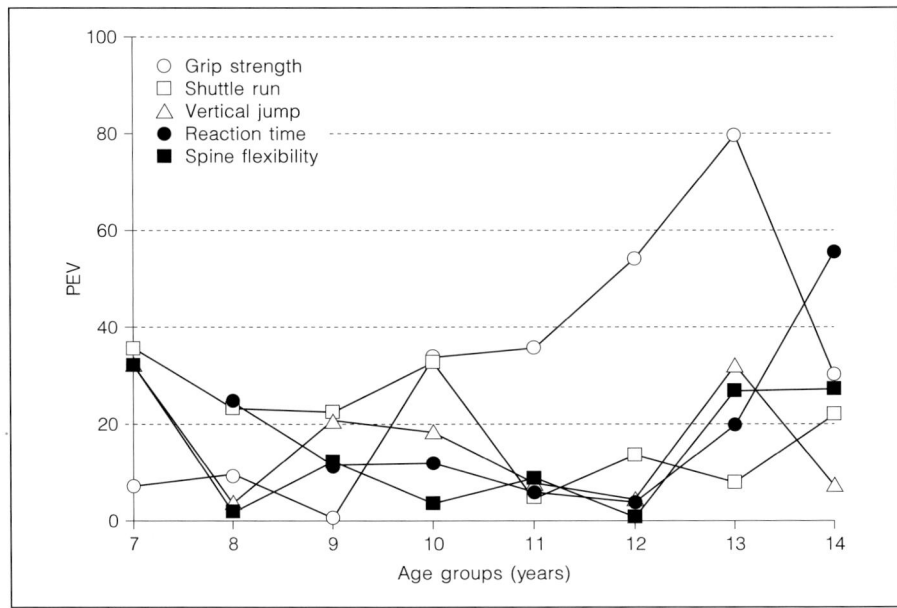

Fig. 4. PEV in physical fitness variables explained by the regression of the anthropometric measurements on each performance task (Polish girls).

mance tasks), do not change significantly with age. These results prove the second hypothesis that physical fitness variables which show significant changes with age during progressive development, as well as being less complex are more dependent on body build parameters. In contrast, other measures are more resistant to change with age and are more functionally complex.

Summary and Conclusions

The comparison of somatic and physical fitness variables between children from Merida (Mexico) and Łódź (Poland) revealed that Polish children were taller and heavier. For grip strength and vertical jump, Mexican children achieved better results in the earlier years (up to 9 years of age), after which Polish boys displayed greater strength and both sexes performed better in the vertical jump. Results for the shuttle run, reaction time and spine flexibility were generally better in Polish children. A correction for biological age (Łódź children showed 1-year delay in biological development as compared with Merida children) augmented the observed differences in body build and physical fitness variables.

Table 10. Statistically significant differences between Merida (Mexico) and Łódź (Poland) schoolchildren in anthropometric and physical fitness variables

Somatic measures and motor tasks	Age groups of studied children, years							
	7	8	9	10	11	12	13	14
Body height								
Boys								
1	P***	P***	P***	P***	P***	P***	P***	P***
2	P*	P***	P***	P***	P***	P***	P***	P***
Girls								
1	P***	P***	P**	P***	P***	P***	P***	P***
2	P**	P***	P***	P***	P***	P***	P***	P***
Body weight								
Boys								
1	P**	P**	P*				P*	P*
2		P***	P***	P***	P***	P***	P**	P**
Girls								
1							P**	P*
2	P*	P**	P**	P**	P***	P***	P***	P**
Arm circumference								
Boys								
1		P*	P*					
2		P**	P***	P***	P**	P*		
Girls								
1								
2						P*		
Grip strength								
Boys								
1			M**		P***		P*	P**
2					P***	P***	P*	P***
Girls								
1	M***	M*						
2	M**				P**			
Vertical jump index								
Boys								
1		M**			P**			P*
						P***		P**
Girls								
1					P*		P*	P**
2					P*	P**		P**

Table 10 (continued)

Somatic measures and motor tasks	Age groups of studied children, years							
	7	8	9	10	11	12	13	14
Shuttle run								
Boys								
1	P**						P*	P**
2		P***					P**	P***
Girls								
1	P**	P*		P***		P***	P***	P***
2	P*	P***	P**		P***	P***	P***	P***
Spine flexibility index								
Boys								
1	P**	P**	P***					
2	P*	P***	P**	P*		P**		
Girls								
1	P***	P***	P***	P**	P**	P**	P***	P***
2	P***	P***	P***	P***	P**	P**	P***	P***
Reaction time								
Boys								
1							P*	
2				P*	P*			P**
Girls								
1		P***	P**	P*			P*	P*
2			P***	P*	P***		P**	P*

Greater values of somatic variables and better results in physical fitness in Poland (P) or Mexico (M) are indicated. *p < 0.05; **p < 0.01; ***p < 0.001. 1 = Differences according to calendar age; 2 = differences after a 1-year shift of trait values of Merida children into older age.

Grip strength, shuttle run and vertical jump, parameters which changed significantly between age groups, showed greater dependence on body build parameters (stature, weight and arm circumference) than spine flexibility and reaction time. A strong genetic contribution is hypothesized in relation to grip strength and shuttle run. The vertical jump seems to be less genetically controlled, with the weakest genetic determination being expected for spine flexibility and reaction time.

References

1. Pařízková J, Merhautová J: The comparison of somatic development, body composition and functional characteristics in Tunisian and Chech boys of 11 and 12 years. Hum Biol 1970;42:391–400.
2. Malina MR: Kinanthropometric research in human auxology; in Borms J, Hauspie R, Sand A, Susanne C, Hebbelinck M (eds): Human Growth and Development. New York, Plenum Press, 1984, pp 437–451.
3. Szopa J: Physical fitness of boys at the age of 12–18 years from Sfax (Tunisia) compared to their peers from Kraków, considering the level of somatic development (comparative approach). Antropomotoryka 1989;1:65–75.
4. Ignasiak Z, Sławińska T: A relative comparison of development of chosen morphological traits in urban children from Tunisia and Poland. Antropomotoryka 1996;14:41–53.
5. Przewęda R, Trześniowski R: Physical fitness of Polish youth in the light of 1989 studies (in Polish). Studia i Monografie. Warsaw, Akademia Wychowania Fizycznego, 1996.
6. Renson R, Beunen G, De Vitte L, Ostyn M, Simons J, Van Gerven D: The social spectrum of the physical fitness of 12- to 19-year-old boys; in Ostyn M, Beunen G, Simons J (eds): Kinanthropometry. Baltimore, University Park Press, 1980, pp 104–118.
7. Wolański N: Methods of Control and Norms of Development of Children and Youth (in Polish). Warsaw, PZWL, 1975.
8. Malina RM, Moriyama M: Growth and motor performance of black and white children 6–10 years of age: A multivariate analysis. Am J Hum Biol 1991;3:599–611.
9. Siniarska A: Physical fitness in Polish population (genetics and development); in Wolański N, Siniarska A (eds): Genetics of Psychomotor Traits in Man. Warsaw, International Society of Sport Genetics and Somatology, 1984, pp 167–188.
10. Szopa J, Mleczko E: Longitudinal family studies on genetic conditioning of functional traits in boys and girls between seven and fourteen. Antropomotoryka 1992;7:11–29.
11. Szopa J: Genetic determinations of motor capability – A problem review (in Polish). Antropomotoryka 1992;8:141–155.
12. Wolański N, Dickinson F, Siniarska A: Seasonal rhythm of menarche as a sensitive index of living conditions. Stud Hum Ecol 1993;11:171–191.
13. Hulanicka B, Brajczewski C, Jedlińska W, Sławińska T, Waliszko A: City – Town – Village, Growth of Children in Poland in 1988. Monographs of the Institute of Anthropology. Wrocław, Polish Academy of Sciences, 1990, p 7.
14. Przewęda R, Wolański N: The relation of economic and demographic conditions to body build and motor fitness in Polish youth; in Pařízková J, Douglas PP (eds): Human Growth, Dietary Intake, and Other Environmental Factors. Proceeding of a Symposium. 13th International Congress of Anthropological and Ethnological Sciences. Mexico City, Institut Danone, 1993, pp 63–71.
15. Wolański N, Pařízková J: Physical Fitness and Human Development (in Polish). Warsaw, Sport i Turystyka, 1976.
16. Orvanová E: Body build heredity and sport achievements; in Wolański N, Siniarska A (eds): Genetics of Psychomotor Traits in Man. Warsaw, International Society of Sport Genetics and Somatology, 1984, pp 111–123.

Dr. Anna Siniarska, CINVESTAV-Merida, Km. 6 Ant. Carr a Progreso,
AP Cordemex, CP 97310, Merida, Yucatan (Mexico)
Tel: +52 99 81 29 20, Fax: +52 99 81 46 70, E-Mail ania@kin.cieamer.conacyt.mx

Dr. Anna Jeziorek, Dr. Maria Nowakowska, Department of Physical Education and Health,
Łódź University, ul. Rudzka 56, PL-93-423 Łódź (Poland)

Body Composition, Body Satisfaction, Eating and Exercise Behavior of Australian Adolescents

Andrew P. Hills, Nuala M. Byrne

School of Human Movement Studies, Queensland University of Technology, Brisbane, Australia

Cardiovascular Health of Australian Children and Adolescents

An awareness of cardiovascular risk factors in adulthood has been commonplace in health promotion for some time, but the importance of primary prevention in childhood and adolescence, and the tracking of risk factors in these populations has been a more recent consideration [1, 2].

Body fat, blood pressure, physical (in)activity and diet can have an individual effect on health status but there are often interactions between these factors. For example, Milligan et al. [3] used a population-specific form of cluster analysis and identified that approximately one fifth of 15-year-old West Australian schoolchildren possessed a range of unhealthy life-style factors which placed them at a substantial risk of cardiovascular disease and other ill health later in life.

Body composition is an extremely important indicator of health status in children and adolescents. The level of body fatness is routinely used to examine the risk of hypertension, insulin-dependent diabetes mellitus and obesity in youths. Bermingham et al. [4] examined the effects of smoking, physical activity and body mass index on total cholesterol (TC) and high-density lipoprotein cholesterol (HDL-C) and found that physical activity was associated with a lower atherogenic TC/HDL-C ratio and that girls with a body mass index (BMI) greater than the 90th centile had higher mean TC/HDL-C and apoprotein B levels than the group as a whole.

It is well recognized that appropriate levels of body weight and adiposity are related to good health, and that obesity is associated with cardiorespiratory, articular, social and psychological complications. Dwyer and Blizzard [5] investigated the association of fatness in children with dyslipoproteinemia and high blood pressure and suggested that the biomedical status of individual children be used to define criteria for obesity. A cutoff of 30% body mass as fat for girls and 20% for boys was deemed an appropriate standard.

The coexistence of multiple cardiovascular risk factors and poor dietary patterns led Milligan et al. [3], to describe the occurrence as similar to the syndrome X of dyslipidemia, hypertension, hyperinsulinemia and insulin resistance, and obesity. The same research group [6], in a controlled trial involving over 1,000 10- to 12-year-old children, found that fitness was improved by physical activity programs which were also associated with a greater fall in diastolic blood pressure and triceps skinfolds in girls compared to controls. The group [7] concluded that higher risk children showed greater responses to life-style intervention, with greatest effects seen with home nutrition or fitness programs.

A large proportion of the Australian adult population is inactive. Thirty-two percent are sedentary and 36% exercise infrequently or at very low energy levels [8]. Unfortunately, the same type of information is not available for children and adolescents. School-based daily physical activity programs were employed in parts of Australia many years ago [9] but were not sustained. Interestingly, there has been a heightened interest in the value of such school-based activity, but there is still an urgent need for a better understanding of the physical activity levels of Australian children [10]. The last reported survey of the physical activity and fitness status of a large sample of Australian schoolchildren was conducted in the mid-1980s [11]. Whilst the completion of a large study of approximately 5,500 adolescents is imminent, there is no representative longitudinal data to quantify the probable decline in levels of physical activity of Australians from childhood through to adulthood in recent times.

Overweight and Obesity in Australian Children and Adolescents

As is the case in many other countries, overweight and obesity are not limited to the Australian adult population. There have been numerous but varying reports of the prevalence of overfatness in childhood and adolescence, but measurement in the younger age groups can be difficult. Indicators have included 120% of ideal weight, BMI percentiles and skinfolds. Estimates based on 120% of a standard or reference weight have concluded that the prevalence of overweight in Australian children is 25–30% but this approach has been criticized due to the failure to adjust for age.

Earlier work of Hills and Parker [12, 13] and Hills [14] consistently used the 95th percentile weight for age as a cutoff for obesity as did Himes and

Table 1. Prevalence of 'overweight' and 'at risk of overweight' in Australian children aged 9–15 years included in the 1985 Australian health and fitness survey

Age years	Sample size	BMI 85th percentile criteria[a]	Proportion at risk of overweight (1985)[b] %	BMI 95th percentile criteria[a]	Proportion overweight (1985)[c] %
Males					
9	482	18.9	10.8	21.5	4.8
10	493	19.6	9.9	22.2	3.0
11	489	20.3	11.2	23.1	5.3
12	494	21.0	9.7	23.9	5.9
13	466	21.6	10.9	24.7	4.3
14	467	22.2	11.6	25.7	3.4
15	451	22.8	11.5	26.6	3.5
All ages	3,217		10.8		4.3
Females					
9	488	19.1	11.1	20.9	7.2
10	497	19.9	7.8	21.9	5.6
11	484	20.6	11.2	23.2	6.0
12	489	21.5	9.2	23.0	4.3
13	438	22.3	11.4	24.5	6.4
14	408	23.1	5.9	25.0	6.1
15	413	23.9	6.8	25.4	8.2
All ages	3,342		9.1		6.2
Total	6,559		10.0		5.3

Source: NHMRC, 1997.
[a] Lazarus et al. [16] from smoothed age- and gender-specific distributions of BMI.
[b] 85th percentile < BMI < 95th percentile.
[c] BMI ≥ 95th percentile.

Dietz [15]. In keeping with trends in the US [15], Lazarus et al. [16] have suggested that the more stable 85th percentile be used to classify those 'at risk' of overweight (see table 1). A study by Harvey and Althaus [17], using the 1985 data set of schoolchildren [11], identified that the 95th percentile in Australian children was lower than in the US. From these data, 5.3% of the children would have been overweight and a further 10% at risk of overweight.

Whilst the BMI has been widely used as an indicator of obesity in epidemiological studies of adults, it cannot distinguish weight from fatness. In relation to children and adolescents, longer-term data linking BMI as a child to obesity and its morbidity in adulthood is not available. Further, the lack of consensus in the literature regarding appropriate descriptors for levels of overfatness has been a major shortcoming and means that prevalence values in absolute terms for children and adolescents are not available at this time [10].

A recent initiative of the National Health and Medical Research Council (NHMRC) was to develop a strategic plan for the prevention of overweight and obesity. Concerned with increased levels of fatness, concomitant with inactivity and poor dietary practices, a working party of the NHMRC proposed national physical activity strategies [10]. Key examples of categories include the development of national guidelines for physical activity which recognize the importance of incidental activity and low to moderate activity. The promotion and implementation of these guidelines includes the incorporation of daily physical activity in school programs. In conjunction, key recommendations have been proposed for dietary improvements. The focus of the recommendations for children and adolescents in the strategic plan [10] is to encourage young people to be physically active, enjoy a wide range of physical activities, continue to be physically active as they get older, consume a healthy diet, and develop skills that will enable them to select, prepare and consume a healthy diet as they get older.

Size and Shape: Perceptions and Behaviors

In the recent past, there has been an increasing preoccupation of many individuals with body weight, diet and exercise [18, 19]. Emphasis on physical fitness and leanness has resulted in a heightened concern with body shape in both sexes, but particularly in girls [20, 21]. The weight control practices employed by males and females appear to reflect this concern [22–26].

The common sociocultural expectation that one attain an 'ideal' body shape has magnified to the extent that some individuals struggle to achieve unrealistic ectomorphic proportions. Exercise participation and dietary modification are the primary strategies cited in attempts to alter body shape and weight [27]. In parallel, there has been a considerable amount of research devoted to the assessment of appearance-related body image, weight control practices, and eating disorders [28, 29].

The most prevalent theory regarding gender differences in appearance-related body image is that males are more satisfied than females with physical appearance [20]. There is clear evidence that the adult preoccupation with weight has extended to child and adolescent populations [26, 30, 31]. Tiggerman and Pennington [20] have reported that 9- and 10-year-old children typically prefer a thinner body than their own.

Unfortunately, variability in the assessment protocols employed has meant that the interpretation of results in the area reflects as much the assessment methodology used as the data collected [31]. Research with adult populations is predominant with little consideration of age and gender differences across the childhood and adolescent years. There have been fewer examples of studies that have linked body morphology (size, shape and composition) and satisfaction with physical appearance. This important area will form the basis of the balance of this chapter with recent research work by the authors presented and discussed.

A Study of the Anthropometric, Status, Body Image and Weight Control Practices of Australian Adolescents

Rationale

Studies with adult populations indicate that preoccupation with body weight and shape is often reflected in the adoption of restrictive dietary practices and other harmful methods of weight regulation [25]. It is evident that such concerns have extended to child and adolescent populations [30, 32, 33]. Cognizant of the increasing societal pressure on adolescents of both sexes to meet the 'ideal' physique, the current study sought to ascertain the level of body fat and physical characteristics of adolescents, and relate this to appearance and weight control attitudes and behaviors (table 2).

Body Image

Body image is a multidimensional construct including both self-perceptual and subjective components [34]. A disturbed body image can result from a subjective evaluation that the body does not meet the perceived ideal, referred to as body dissatisfaction [35]. Whilst it has been well documented that a disturbance in body image is often associated with a desire to alter physical appearance in adults [18, 28, 34], less research has addressed this relationship across the adolescent years.

Body Satisfaction

Comparable with findings of adult studies, male adolescents in the current study were significantly more satisfied than females with their physical appearance in general, and with weight-related aspects in particular. Although males were more satisfied, the majority of both sexes (79.5% males, 83.7% females) indicated that if given the opportunity they would alter their physique in some way. However, the direction of the desired change differed between the sexes. More than twice as many females (70.4%) as males (34.4%) indicated a desire

Table 2. Physical characteristics of subjects

	Male (n = 122)			Female (n = 95)		
	mean	SD	range	mean	SD	range
Age, years	14.5	0.6	13–15	14.7	0.5	13–15
Height, cm	166.9	8.5	148.1–185.7	162.4	6.6	147.6–172.9
Weight, kg	56.7	10.8	32.4–83.4	54.7	9.7	33.9–80.2
BMI	20.2	2.9	14.8–28.6	20.7	3.8	15.3–35.7
Endomorphy	3.3	1.7	1.5–8.8	4.4	1.5	2.3–9.6
Mesomorphy	4.8	1.3	2.2–9.0	4.1	1.5	1.7–9.6
Ectomorphy	3.4	1.4	0.1–6.3	3.0	1.5	0.1–6.1
Skinfolds[a]	92.3	49.7	43.5–260.4	125.5	45.1	63.1–310.4

[a] Sum of 8 skinfolds (mm; triceps, subscapular, biceps, iliac crest, supraspinale, abdominal, front thigh, medial calf).

to be thinner. In contrast, more males (45.1%) than females (13.3%) reported a desire for a larger physique. Therefore, although both male and female adolescents were less satisfied with a physique displaying a higher level of adiposity, males wished to be more muscular, while females desired to be thinner. In a recent study by O'Dea et al. [32], 66.7% of participants, aged 11.1–14.7 years, perceived their body weight to be satisfactory. In general, this study indicated that more males perceived themselves as too thin and more females felt they were too fat.

Smolak et al. [30] have reported an association between puberty and an increase in body dissatisfaction in females. The results of this study suggest that the onset of puberty may influence body satisfaction for both sexes. Earlier research identified that males and females 9–10 years of age do not differ significantly in their level of body satisfaction [20]. Results of the current study demonstrated evidence of a significant gender difference at 12 years of age, with females displaying a marked level of body dissatisfaction while males were satisfied with their physical appearance. The relationship between body image and self-concept is much higher for females than males at this age, and has been attributed to the onset of puberty for females around the age of 12 [36]. The current study found that males 14 years of age displayed a level of dissatisfaction with their physical appearance comparable with their female peers. This decrease in body satisfaction for males coincides with the age at which males, on average, begin puberty [37].

Results from other research [38] has shown that the gender difference reemerged by 16 years of age, with males reporting satisfaction as they progress towards the adult physique, in contrast to females who remained dissatisfied. Thus, the onset of puberty does appear to be associated with a marked level of body dissatisfaction for both sexes.

The Influence of Body Composition on Weight Control Practices

It appears that current body size influences body satisfaction to some extent. A higher weight-for-height ratio, and higher adiposity levels were associated with lower body satisfaction for both male and female adolescents. Those with a higher level of adiposity thought and felt they were larger than their peers who displayed less adiposity. The gender differences in body and weight satisfaction noted above were not evident in comparing adolescent males and females with lower levels of adiposity. In addition, when normalized for weight for height, females were no more likely to perceive themselves as overweight. These results suggest that due to its centrality to physical appearance, body weight and level of adiposity are fundamental elements of physical attractiveness standards for both sexes.

Inappropriate weight control attempts can have maladaptive long-term consequences such as the adoption of disordered eating practices, growth retardation, delayed menarche, amenorrhea, osteoporosis and psychological disturbances [39–42]. Weight control practices in modern society such as dietary modification and exercise are pervasive, whether for health or esthetic reasons.

In support of previous research on adolescents [27, 43], females in the current study were significantly more likely than males to diet (61 vs. 8.0%) and fast (18.9 vs. 1.8%) for weight control. Female adolescents were also more likely to employ pathogenic weight control practices, and count the energy content of foods consumed. As there is great diversity in the reported prevalence of weight control practices of both adult and adolescent populations, it is difficult to assess the normalcy of these results for the male and female adolescents tested. However, the prevalence of dieting and fasting are within the range of results reported elsewhere [27, 42], and support the supposition that dieting to address preoccupations with weight and physical appearance may be considered normative for females [29, 44, 45]. The gender differences in weight-related concerns and practices may be attributed to the fact that while a similar proportion of males and females (8.9 and 10.5%, respectively) were considered overweight, nearly twice as many females as males (25.3 vs. 13.4%) perceived themselves to be overweight. However, more importantly, 72% of females in contrast to 28% of males reported 'feeling fat'. Overestimation of weight in normal-weight subjects is commonly in the range 30–36% [21]. In a study of families with an adolescent aged 14–15 years, Tienboon et al. [46] found that 41% of girls and 14% of boys considered themselves overweight. In this group, 18% of both boys and girls were overweight on the basis of BMI. As suggested by Killen et al. [33], the heightened concern of females in particular, with weight-related aspects of the body, appears to be well-established by adolescence. This is the case despite the fact that a comparable proportion of males and females are considered overweight. According to Striegel-Moore et al. [45], adolescent females' concerns with body weight are due to their equating 'normal' weight with 'underweight'. This would reflect an ignorance of the appropriate body weight for their age, skeletal size, and muscularity. Alternatively, as suggested by Koff and Rierdan [36], these females are aware of appropriate weight norms, however deliberately they try to violate them, reflecting dissatisfaction with body weight.

There was no gender difference in the weekly frequency of exercise participation between the sexes, due most probably to compulsory sport and physical activity sessions at school. However, there were differences in the exercise motivations males and females reported. Females were more likely to exercise for appearance/weight management, to improve muscle tone, and for stress/mood management. Male adolescents were more likely to exercise for health/fitness-related reasons.

Consistent with previous findings [19, 43], motivations for exercise activity such as weight control, tone, and attractiveness were associated with increased body dissatisfaction and restricting tendencies (drive-for-thinness) for females in particular. In contrast, those individuals motivated to exercise for fitness, health and enjoyment were less likely to report disturbances in body satisfaction and eating-related attitudes and behaviors. Consequently, as suggested by McDonald and Thompson [19], there is cause for concern for elevated eating dysfunction and body dissatisfaction in individuals, particularly females, who report that they exercise for reasons associated with body weight, muscle tone, and/or attractiveness.

Conclusion

In recent years there has been a more concerted effort to utilize methodology to assess the relationships between body composition and health-related behaviors. However, whilst more research is required to gain a full appreciation of these relationships, and how they may influence health in the longer term, it is clear that body composition, weight control behaviors and health status are associated from an early age.

References

1 Gliksman MD, Dwyer T, Boulton TJC: Should the primary prevention of coronary heart disease commence in childhood? Med J Aust 1987;146:360–362.
2 World Health Organisation: Prevention in childhood and youth of adult cardiovascular disease: Time for action. WHO Technical Report Series. Geneva, WHO,1990, No 792.
3 Milligan RA, Thompson C, Vandongen R, Beilin LJ, Burke V: Clustering of cardiovascular risk factors in Australian adolescents: Association with dietary excesses and deficiencies. J Cardiovasc Risk 1996;2:515–523.
4 Bermingham MA, Jones E, Steinbeck K, Brock K: Plasma cholesterol and other cardiac risk factors in adolescent girls. Arch Dis Child 1995;73(suppl 5):392–397.
5 Dwyer T, Blizzard CL: Defining obesity in children by biological endpoint rather than population distribution. Int J Obes 1996;20(suppl 5):472–480.
6 Burke V, Beilin LJ, Milligan R, Thompson C: An assessment of nutrition and physical activity education programs in children. Clin Exp Pharmacol Physiol 1995;22:212–216.
7 Beilin L, Burke V, Milligan R: Strategies for prevention of adult hypertension and cardiovascular risk behaviour in childhood. An Australian perspective. J Hum Hypertens 1996;10(suppl 1):S51–S54.
8 National Heart Foundation: National Heart Foundation Risk Factor Study No 3 1989. Canberra, NHF and AIHW, 1990.
9 Dwyer T, Coonan WE, Leitch DR, Hetzel BS, Baghurst PA: An investigation of the effects of daily physical activity on the health of primary school children in South Australia. Int J Epidemiol 1983; 2:303–313.
10 National Health and Medical Research Council: Acting on Australia's Weight. Canberra, Australian Government Publishing Service, 1997.
11 Pyke JE: Australian Health and Fitness Survey 1985: The Fitness, Health and Physical Performance of Australian School Students aged 7–15 years. Parkside, ACHPER,1987.
12 Hills AP, Parker AW: Obesity management via diet and exercise intervention. Child Care Health Dev 1988;14:409–416.
13 Hills AP, Parker AW: Anthropometric and body composition assessment of obese children. J Sports Sci 1990;8/2:175–176.
14 Hills AP: Effects of diet and exercise on body composition of pre-pubertal children. J Phys Educ Sports Sci 1991;3/2:22–26.
15 Himes JH, Dietz WH: Guidelines for overweight in adolescent preventive services: Recommendations from an expert committee. Am J Clin Nutr 1994;59:307–316.
16 Lazarus R, Baur L, Webb K, Blyth F, Gliksman M: Recommended body mass index cut-off values for overweight screening programmes in Australian children and adolescents: Comparisons with North American values. J Paediatr Child Health 1995;31:143–147.
17 Harvey PWJ, Althaus MA: The distribution of body mass index in Australian children aged 7–15 years. Aust J Nutr Diet 1993;50:151–153.
18 Brownell KD, Rodin J, Wilmore JH: Eating, body weight and performance in athletes: An introduction; in Brownell KD, Rodin J, Wilmore JH (eds): Eating, Body Weight and Performance. London, Lea & Febiger, 1992, pp 3–14.
19 McDonald K, Thompson JK: Eating disturbance, body image dissatisfaction, and reasons for exercising: Gender differences and correlational findings. Int J Eat Disord 1992;11/3:289–292.
20 Tiggerman M, Pennington B: The development of gender differences in body-size satisfaction. Aust Psych 1990;41:246–263.
21 Paxton SJ, Wertheim EH, Gibbons K, Szmukler GI, Hillier L, Petrovich J: Body image satisfaction, dieting belief and weight loss behaviours in adolescent girls and boys. J Youth Adolesc 1991;20: 361–379.
22 Maude D, Wertheim EH, Paxton S, Gibbons K, Szmukler G: Body dissatisfaction, weight loss behaviours and bulimic tendencies in Australian adolescents with an estimate of female data representativeness. Aust Psych 1993;28/2:128–132.
23 Nowak M, Speare R, Crawford D: Gender differences in adolescent weight and shape related beliefs and behaviours. J Paediatr Child Health 1996;32:148–152.

24 O'Dea J: Food habits, body image and self-esteem of adolescent girls from disadvantaged and non-disadvantaged backgrounds. Aust J Nutr Diet 1994;51:74–78.
25 Rodin J, Larson L: Social factors and the ideal body image, in Brownell KD, Rodin J, Wilmore JH (eds): Eating, Body Weight and Performance in Athletes. London, Lea & Febiger, 1992.
26 Wertheim EH, Paxton SJ, Maude D, Smukler GI, Gibbons K, Hiller L: Psychosocial predictors of weight-loss behaviours and binge eating in adolescent girls and boys. Int J Eat Disord 1992;12/2:151–160.
27 Emmons L: Dieting and purging behavior in black and white highschool students. J Am Diet Assoc 1992;92:306–312.
28 Cooper MJ, Fairburn CG: Thoughts about eating, weight and shape in anorexia nervosa and bulimia nervosa. Behav Res Ther 1992;30:501–511.
29 Koff E, Rierdan J: Perceptions of weight and attitudes toward eating in early adolescent girls. J Adolesc Health 1991;12:307–312.
30 Smolak L, Levine MP, Gralen S: The impact of puberty and dating on eating problems among middle school girls. J Youth Adolesc 1993;22:355–369.
31 Byrne NM, Hills AP: Should body-image scales designed for adults be used with adolescents? Percept Mot Skills 1996;82:747–753.
32 O'Dea J, Abraham S, Heard R: Food habits, body image and weight control practices of young male and female adolescents. Aust J Nutr Diet 1996;53/1:32–38.
33 Killen JD, Taylor CB, Hammer LD, Litt I, Wilson DM, Rich T, Haywood C, Simmonds B, Kraemer H, Varady A: An attempt to modify unhealthful eating attitudes and weight regulation practices of young adolescent girls. Int J Eat Disord 1993;13:369–384.
34 Garfinkel PE, Goldbloom D, Davis R, Olmstead MP, Garner DM, Halmi K: Body dissatisfaction in bulimia nervosa: Relationship to weight and shape concerns and psychological functioning. Int J Eat Disord 1992;11/2:151–161.
35 Garner DM, Garfinkel PE: Body image in anorexia nervosa: Measurement, theory, and clinical implications. Int J Psychiatry Med 1981;11:263–284.
36 Koff E, Rierdan J, Stubbs M: Gender, body image, and self-concept in early adolescence J Early Adolesc 1990;10/1:56–68.
37 Malina RM, Bouchard C: Growth, Maturation and Physical Activity. Champaign, Human Kinetics, 1991.
38 Byrne NM, Hills AP: Assessment of eating practices in adolescence. Proc Nutr Soc (Aust) 1995; 19:106.
39 Carbon RJ: Exercise, amenorrhoea and the skeleton. Br Med J 1992;48:546–560.
40 Davis C, Fox J: Excessive exercise and weight preoccupation in women. Addict Behav 1993;18:201–211.
41 Treble GF, Morton AR: A recipe for success or tragedy? Selection for Australian Rhythmic Gymnastic Representation. Sports Health 1994;12/2:5–10.
42 Greenfeld D, Quinlan D, Harding M, Glass E, Bliss A: Eating behaviour in an adolescent population. Int J Eat Disord 1987;6/1:99–111.
43 Silberstein L, Striegel-Moore R, Timko C, Rodin J: Behavioral and psychological implications of body dissatisfaction: Do men and women differ? Sex Roles 1988;19:219–232.
44 Mellin LM, Irwin CE, Scully S: Prevalence of disordered eating in girls: A survey of middle-class children. JAMA 1992;92:851–853.
45 Striegel-Moore RH, Silberstein LR, Rodin J: Toward an understanding of risk factors for bulimia. Am Psychol 1986;41:246–263.
46 Tienboon P, Rutishauser IH, Wahlqvist ML: Adolescents' perception of body weight and parents' weight for height status. J Adolesc Health 1994;15(suppl 3):263–268.

Associate Professor A.P. Hills, School of Human Movement Studies,
Queensland University of Technology, Victoria Park Road,
Brisbane, Kelvin Grove, QLD 4059 (Australia)

Sex Differences in Physical Fitness in Flemish Youth

J. Lefevre[a], *G. Beunen*[a], *J. Borms*[b], *J. Vrijens*[c]

[a] Centre for Physical Development Research, Faculty of Physical Education and Physiotherapy, KU Leuven,
[b] Laboratory of Human Biometry, Faculty of Physical Education and Physical Therapy, Vrije Universiteit Brussel, and
[c] Institute of Physical Education, Universiteit Gent, Belgium

Introduction

Generally, most physical performance capacities improve with age during childhood and adolescence. Moreover, during this life period sex differences are observed for a variety of physical performance tasks. However, since the tempo and timing of the growth patterns of both sexes are not the same, the differences are not so marked at all ages and during some periods of the growth process, the differences are even reversed.

An excellent overview of results concerning sexual dimorphism in physical performance has been put together by Malina and Bouchard [1]. As a summary, it can be concluded that on average, the motor performance of girls reaches a plateau and may decline during adolescence, whereas strength increases slowly with age during adolescence. In contrast, the strength and motor performance of boys generally increase during adolescence resulting in significant differences.

Explanations of gender differences can be sought in biological and environmental factors, and their interaction. Biology seems to offer little explanation for motor performance differences prior to puberty; differences are primarily environmentally induced. However, biology does appear to play a greater role in gender differences during adolescence [2].

The purpose of this study was to document differences between male and female Flemish youngsters with test scores from the EUROFIT test battery

Table 1. Number of subjects used in the analyses per age group for each sex and in total

Age group	Boys	Girls	Total
6	178	197	375
7	223	314	537
8	213	271	484
9	285	306	591
10	275	327	602
11	364	401	765
12	610	617	1,227
13	552	521	1,073
14	425	510	935
15	448	457	905
16	441	486	927
17	379	382	711
18	169	122	291
Total	4,562 (48)	4,921 (52)	9,483

Figures in parentheses represent percentage.

and to examine one aspect of the biological explanation, that is to determine the contribution of height, weight and subcutaneous fat to sex differences in physical fitness.

Materials and Methods

Subjects

The data are derived from a cross-sectional survey of the physical fitness of a representative sample of 9,483 Flemish boys and girls, 6–18 years of age. All subjects were investigated between 1989 and 1993 during the normal school period. A multistage, proportional cluster sampling procedure was used. In the first stage, a proportionate, stratified sample with schools as the primary sampling clusters was selected. The different strata were selected according to the structure of the Flemish school system and the geographical distribution of the schools. The sample included primary as well as secondary schools. In the second stage, entire classes of boys and/or girls were selected from the 12 grades in the schools. The final sample consisted of approximately 48% boys and 52% girls. Subjects were classified according to age (see table 1).

Measurements and Tests

The primary purpose of this survey was to evaluate the physical fitness status of Flemish youths, using EUROFIT, the European test of physical fitness. Somatic measurements as well as different motor characteristics were included. The somatic measurements comprised height, weight and five skinfold sites (triceps, biceps, subscapular, suprailiac and medial calf). As a general measurement of subcutaneous fatness, the sum of the five skinfold sites was calculated.

The battery of fitness tests included four health-related items: (1) sit and reach – flexibility, (2) sit-ups – trunk strength/abdominal muscular endurance, (3) bent-arm hang – functional strength/upper body muscular endurance and (4) endurance shuttle run test – cardiorespiratory endurance, and five performance-related fitness tests: (1) flamingo balance – general balance, (2) plate tapping – speed of limb movement, (3) standing broad jump – explosive strength, (4) hand grip – static strength and (5) shuttle run, 50 m – running speed/agility. A detailed description of each test and the specific protocol is described in the EUROFIT handbook [3]. Average growth curves for both sexes, growth standards and profile charts for each age group and gender were constructed for each of the somatic and performance characteristics [4, 5].

Statistical Analysis

At each age level the sex differences in somatic and motor characteristics were determined using independent Student's t tests. An alpha level of 0.01 was used for all statistical tests. To verify whether somatic characteristics contribute to the explanation of the variance in motor fitness, stepwise multiple regressions were carried out at each age for each of the fitness components as the dependent variables and height, weight and subcutaneous fatness as the independent variables. Based on these results, the differences between boys and girls for the motor fitness tests were reanalyzed by means of an analysis of covariance. To remove the influence of body size differences, the somatic characteristics that explained a significant portion of the variance in the fitness tests were selected as covariates.

Results

Comparisons of the boys and girls are shown in figures 1–3 for somatic characteristics, health-related fitness and motor fitness, respectively. As expected, boys and girls had similar height and weight dimensions until 10 years and thereafter, girls had larger dimensions than boys. From 14 years onwards, boys were significantly taller and from 15 years onwards, they were also significantly heavier. Girls had higher skinfold values than boys throughout the age range and the differences were marked from 13 years of age.

Boys obtained better results at all age levels for cardiorespiratory endurance (endurance shuttle run) and functional strength (bent arm hang) and the differences became more marked after 12 years of age. Boys and girls did not differ significantly at ages 6, 7 and 9 for trunk strength (sit-ups). From age 10 onwards, however, the boys performed significantly better and the differences became greater with increasing age. On the other hand, girls had better flexibility at all ages.

The growth curves for static strength (hand grip) and explosive strength (standing broad jump) show approximately the same pattern but with boys

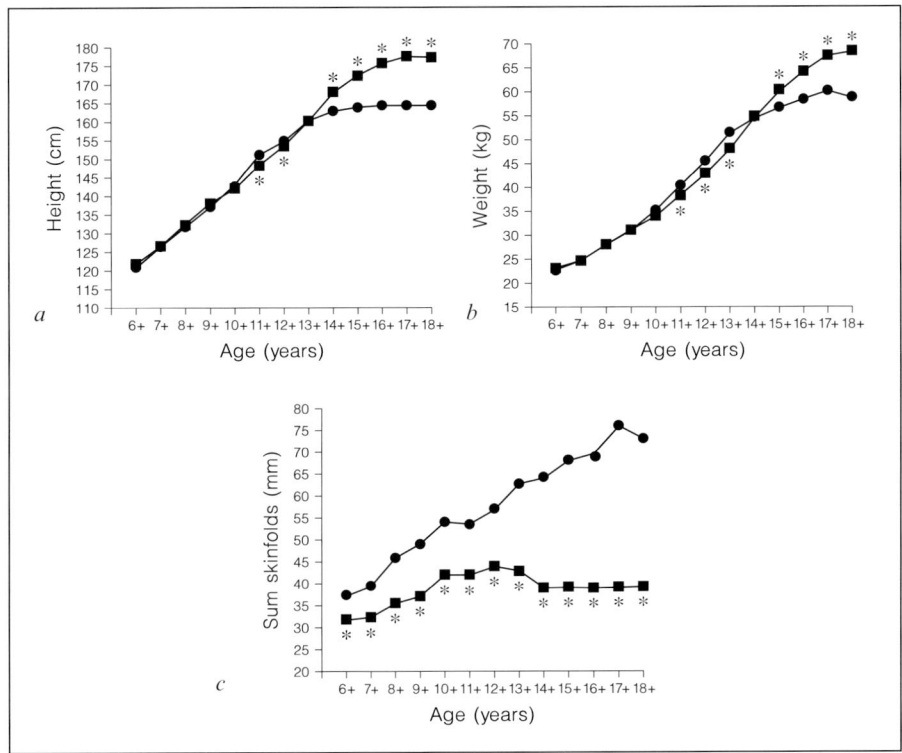

Fig. 1. Height (*a*), weight (*b*) and sum skinfolds (*c*) of Flemish boys (■) and girls (●). *p<0.01 vs. girls.

having superior results. Differences are small between 6 and 12 years of age but beyond 12 there is a linear increase in the mean differences. For running speed (shuttle run), boys were significantly faster. There were no substantial differences between sexes in plate tapping and the flamingo balance test.

The results of the stepwise multiple regressions are given in table 2. For each motor characteristic at each age, the percentages of explained variance are reported with the indication of the somatic characteristics that entered significantly the stepwise regression procedure.

For flexibility (sit and reach), speed of limb movement (plate tapping) and general balance (flamingo balance), the results indicate that only a small portion of the variance can be explained by the interindividual differences in height, weight and subcutaneous fatness. For sit and reach, and plate tapping, no more than 10% of the variance can be explained while for flamingo balance, the highest percentage (15%) was noted at the age of 13. For cardiorespiratory

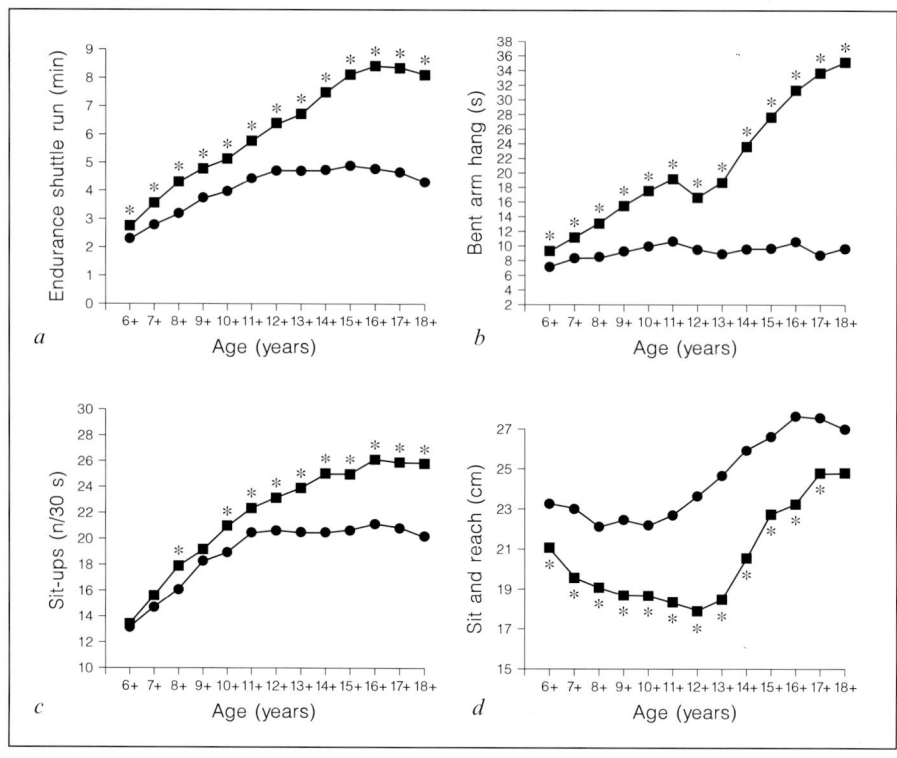

Fig. 2. Performance on health-related fitness tests in Flemish boys (■) and girls (●): cardiorespiratory endurance (*a*), functional strength (*b*), trunk strength (*c*) and flexibility (*d*). *$p<0.01$ vs. girls.

endurance, the different strength tests and for running speed, a substantial portion of the variance can be explained by the somatic characteristics. In general, the 'influence' of the somatic characteristics becomes progressively more important with increasing age. For the endurance shuttle run, bent arm hang, sit-ups, standing broad jump and shuttle run, the variable which enters first into the regression is the sum of skinfolds. All regression coefficients are negative except for the shuttle run. For this test, however, high individual scores point to a poor relative performance. For the most part, weight enters as a second variable.

The highest percentage of explained variance was found for static strength (hand grip). From age 14 onwards, more than 60% can be explained. The most important variable is weight with positive regression coefficients, followed by the sum of skinfolds with negative regression coefficients.

Table 2. Percentages of explained variance for all motor characteristics

Age group	Endurance shuttle run	Bent arm hang	Sit-ups	Sit and reach	Hand grip	Standing broad jump	Shuttle run	Plate tapping	Flamingo balance
6	12 (S+W)	12 (S)	7 (S+H)	–	22 (W+S)	13 (S+W)	10 (S+W)	2 (H)	3 (S)
7	16 (S+W)	12 (S)	8 (S+W)	3 (H+W)	23 (W+S)	19 (S+W+H)	10 (S+W)	9 (H+W)	2 (S)
8	23 (S+W)	16 (S+W)	16 (S+H)	3 (H+W+S)	27 (W+S)	32 (S+W+H)	15 (S+W)	2 (H)	6 (S)
9	27 (S+W)	21 (S)	16 (S+H)	1 (H)	24 (W+S)	29 (S+W)	13 (S+W)	2 (H)	9 (S)
10	29 (S+W)	24 (S+H+W)	20 (S)	–	32 (W+S)	30 (S+W+H)	15 (S+W)	1 (H)	11 (S)
11	27 (S+W+H)	25 (S+H+W)	19 (S+W)	3 (W+H+S)	39 (W+S)	29 (S+W+H)	15 (S+W)	4 (H)	11 (S+W)
12	31 (S+W+H)	30 (S+H)	20 (S+W+H)	3 (W+H+S)	45 (W+S)	30 (S+W)	16 (S+W+H)	3 (H)	11 (S+W)
13	38 (S+W)	30 (S)	25 (S+W)	6 (W+H+S)	52 (W+S)	43 (S+W)	22 (S+W)	5 (W+S)	15 (S+H)
14	41 (S+W+H)	32 (S+W)	26 (S+W+H)	5 (H+W)	59 (W+S)	42 (S+W)	21 (S+W+H)	1 (H)	11 (S+W)
15	49 (S+W)	44 (S+W)	32 (S+W)	3 (H+W)	64 (W+S)	55 (S+W+H)	20 (S+W)	6 (S+W)	11 (S+W)
16	49 (S+W)	45 (S+W)	32 (S+W)	7 (H+W)	68 (W+S)	56 (S+W)	21 (S+W)	3 (S+W)	12 (S+W)
17	47 (S+W)	49 (S+H)	33 (S+W+H)	4 (H+W+S)	67 (W+S)	60 (S+W)	32 (S+W)	6 (S+W)	8 (S+H)
18	46 (S+W+H)	51 (S+W)	34 (S+W+H)	7 (H+W+S)	73 (W+S)	65 (S+W)	28 (S+W)	9 (H)	5 (S)

Independent variables are height (H), weight (W) and subcutaneous fatness (S). Somatic characteristics that entered significantly in the different steps are given in parentheses.

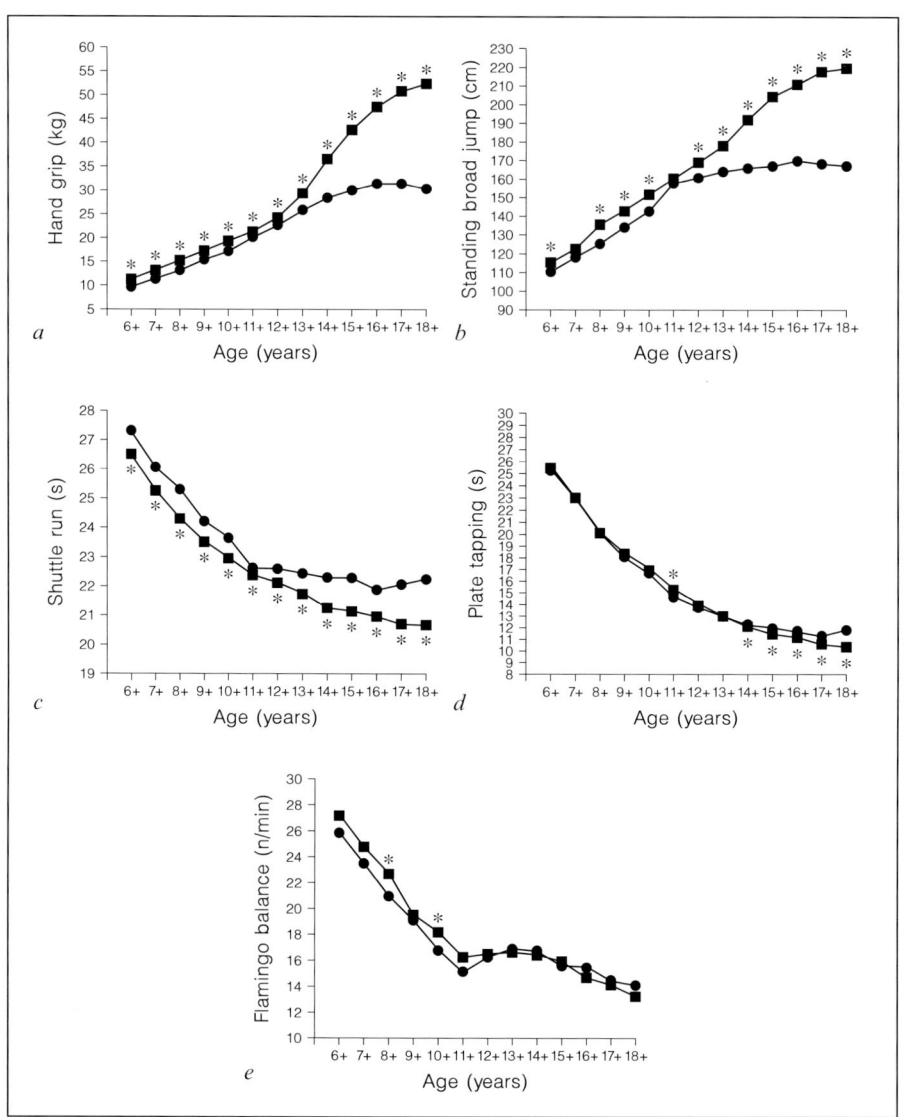

Fig. 3. Performance on motor fitness tests in Flemish boys (■) and girls (●): static strength (*a*), explosive strength (*b*), running speed (*c*), speed of limb movement (*d*) and balance (*e*). *$p < 0.01$ vs. girls.

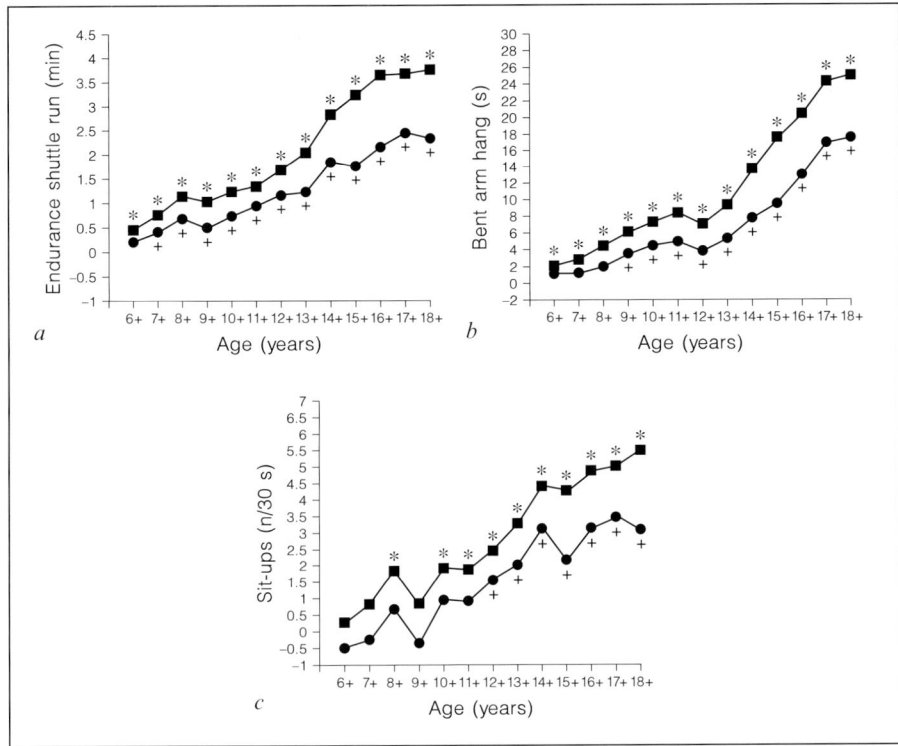

Fig. 4. Differences between the original means of boys and those of girls (■) in comparison with the differences between the ANCOVA-adjusted means of boys and those of girls (●): cardiorespiratory endurance (*a*), functional strength (*b*) and trunk strength (*c*). $^*p<0.01$ before analysis of covariance; $^+p<0.01$ after analysis of covariance.

In figures 4 and 5, the differences between the original means of boys and those of girls are compared with the differences between the ANCOVA-adjusted means of boys and those of girls. Comparisons are only made for the motor characteristics in which a substantial portion of the variance could be explained by the somatic dimensions.

For the endurance shuttle run test, the mean differences are remarkably reduced but are still significantly different from zero (except at the age of 6). The reduction of magnitude of the differences is consistent till the age of 12. After that age, the reductions in the size of differences become much greater. Since the somatic characteristics have a greater influence on functional strength with increasing age (table 2, increasing percentages of explained variance), the adjustments become more important but remain significant. The sex differences

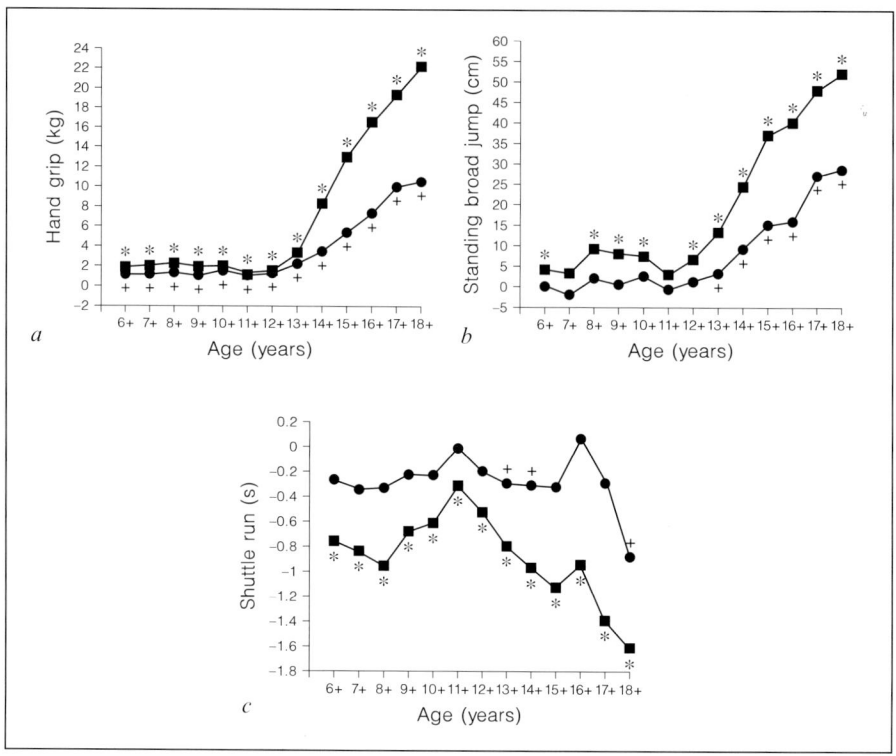

Fig. 5. Differences between the original means of boys and those of girls (■) in comparison with the differences between the ANCOVA-adjusted means of boys and those of girls (●): static strength (*a*), explosive strength (*b*), and running speed (*c*). * $p<0.01$ before analysis of covariance; + $p<0.01$ after analysis of covariance.

between the adjusted means at ages 6–8 years are no more significant. Also for the sit-up test, after analysis of covariance, the sex differences are substantially reduced. No more significant differences were found at the ages of 8, 10 and 11.

The sex differences for static strength remain nearly the same after adjustment for the covariates (weight and subcutaneous fatness) till the age of 13. However, from age 14 onwards, the mean differences between both sexes are reduced with an amount of about 70% although the sex differences between the adjusted means remain significant. After taking into account the 'influence' of the sum of skinfolds and weight and also height at some ages, no more significant differences were noted for the standing broad jump from 6 to 12 years of age. From age 13 onwards, the differences still remain significant (in favor of the boys), but are considerably reduced. Just as for hand grip, during the adolescent age period, the slope of the curve of the differences of the adjusted means is less steep than the curve of the differences of the original means, which indicates that with increasing age, the somatic characteristics have more of an effect on static and explosive strength. Finally, for running speed, all sex differences were significant before the analysis of covariance. After adjustment for the covariates, only significant differences between the means are found at three age groups, 13, 14 and 18 years of age.

Discussion

The curves displayed in figures 1–3 represent age- and sex-specific average distance curves for boys and girls and can be used to evaluate the growth status of children and adolescents but do not portray the wide range of individual variability. Consistent with many previous studies, the height and weight characteristics of both sexes follow the same course of growth. Height shows a linear increase till age 12 for boys and till age 10 for girls. The average growth velocity is approximately 5 cm/year. After this period of linear increase, there is rapid gain during the adolescent spurt. The distance curve for weight shows a more curvilinear increase. During the early part of the adolescent spurt, girls are temporarily taller and heavier due to their earlier growth spurt. At the age of 14 (height) and 15 (weight), on average, boys surpass girls in height and weight. Adult stature is attained, on the average, at age 17 for boys and at age 15 for girls. The highest value for body weight for girls was found at age 17 whilst for boys, body weight continued to increase after age 18. Girls have more subcutaneous fat than boys at all ages. Both curves are parallel between 6 and 11 years of age, in other words the sex differences are constant. From age 12, the growth course of both sexes is completely different. Boys show an increase in subcutaneous fatness from 6 till 12 years of age, followed by a decline through age 14, reaching a plateau at about 40 mm. For girls, however, subcutaneous fat thickness increases almost linearly, except between ages 10 and 11. Sex differences were greater for the skinfolds on the extremities during adolescence than for trunk skinfolds.

For the endurance shuttle run test, both sexes increased linearly from age 6 through age 12. The rate of improvement for boys, however, was higher than for girls, which resulted in greater differences with increasing age. From age 12 onwards, boys continued to increase on average with about 0.5 min/year till age 17, followed by a small decline. Girls, however, showed no more improvement after age 12. The growth curve for bent arm hang for girls showed small increases and mean performances varied between 7 and 11 s. For boys, functional strength improved linearly from 5 to 11 years of age, followed by a small decrease. From 13 years onwards there was a clear spurt, so the sex differences became especially apparent after age 12. At age 18 the mean performance of the boys was more than 3 times the mean performance of the girls. During childhood, the differences in trunk strength are very small, always in favor of the boys. For boys as well as for girls, there was a continuous increase till age 11. From that age onwards, girls showed no more improvement whilst scores for boys increased till age 16. However, as for the bent arm hang test, there was no evidence of a spurt. In contrast to cardiorespiratory endurance and the two muscular endurance tests, girls performed better in flexibility tasks. The mean scores for girls were stable from 6 through 11 years, increased linearly to age 16 and then appeared to reach a plateau. For boys, mean scores declined through age 12, followed by a marked adolescent spurt from age 13 through age 17. The sex difference was greatest during the adolescent spurt of the girls.

The growth curves for the hand grip test and for the standing broad jump have nearly the same pattern. The sex differences in static strength (about 2 kg) and explosive strength (between 5 and 10 cm) are consistent, though small, throughout childhood. Both strength tests increased linearly with age in boys, until 12 years of age for hand grip and until 13 years of age for standing broad jump, followed by an acceleration in strength development. In girls, both strength tests increased linearly with age for about 15 years (hand grip) and about 12 years (standing broad jump). Boys showed a clear adolescent strength spurt, which is not the case for girls. Sex differences therefore become magnified during male adolescence. Running speed improved linearly from 6 through 11 years of age in boys as well as in girls. The slope of the increase was nearly the same in both sexes, resulting in stable differences (about 0.3 s), in favor of the boys. For boys, performance continued to improve at a lesser, but a constant pace, up to 17 years. Girls showed no more improvement in running speed after age 11. Given this plateau in the average performance of girls, the sex difference becomes magnified during adolescence. The performances for speed of limb movement for boys and girls were very similar. The pattern of both growth curves is curvilinear for both sexes, a continuous increase in the mean performance but with a decreased rate of improvement with increasing age. In both sexes, there is a marked linear improvement in balance from 6 through 11 years of age. After that age, girls reach a plateau until age 15, while boys show a decrease in mean performance during the same period. These results equate with some literature [6] that suggests a period of adolescent awkwardness, a temporary disruption of motor coordination during the growth spurt, which is generally attributed to the differential timing of growth spurts of the lower limbs and muscle mass. Data that suggest a plateau or decline in tasks requiring balance at the time of the growth spurt, however, are derived from cross-sectional studies.

Interindividual differences in physical fitness can be explained by a large number of factors. Body size and body composition are important factors that affect performance in both health-related and motor fitness tests. The relationships, however, vary among performance measures and with age. Results in table 2 indicate that body size (height and weight) and subcutaneous fatness have no or little effect on flexibility, speed of limb movement and balance. Explanations of the gender-related difference in flexibility must be sought elsewhere.

Results for the endurance shuttle run test, the different strength tests and for running speed, however, imply a significant role for body size and subcutaneous fatness. From the percentages of explained variance, it is clear that the relationship becomes more important with increasing age. Except for static strength, subcutaneous fatness has the greatest contribution in the explained part of the variance. The regression coefficients were all negative indicating the negative effect of subcutaneous fatness. The greater subcutaneous fatness of girls (see fig. 1c) and also the sex differences in weight and height during adolescence appear to play an important role in gender differences for cardiorespiratory endurance, functional strength, trunk strength and running speed at all ages and especially during the adolescent years for static strength and explosive strength. The differences between the ANCOVA-adjusted means were for most tests substantially reduced resulting in no more significant sex differences during childhood for trunk strength, explosive strength and running speed. When sex differences were controlled for subcutaneous fatness, weight and height, boys still performed significantly better during adolescence in all strength tests as well as regarding cardiorespiratory endurance. Therefore, other factors are probably responsible for the sex differences in some performance and health-related fitness tests of adolescents.

Boys and girls differ in physiological, biochemical and endocrinological characteristics which undoubtedly influence physical fitness. As a result of the production of increasing amounts of testosterone during puberty, boys have more lean body mass than girls and thus in strength tests, adolescent boys have a biological advantage. Since girls attain biological maturity much earlier than boys, it can be expected that girls also attain an earlier plateau in different fitness components.

Social (social pressure to conform) and motivational factors should also be considered, especially in adolescent girls. Sex differences in physical activity and role patterns may contribute to sex differences in physical fitness. The level of sport participation of Flemish girls is significantly lower than that of Belgian boys [7]. As adult women, females change their interest in and attitudes toward physical activity [8], which can partly explain the decrease in cardiorespiratory endurance from age 15 onwards.

Summary and Conclusions

The growth curves for height and weight in Flemish boys and girls in the current population do not differ from other populations. No sexual differences are noted between the ages of 6 and 10. After the well-known 'crossing-over' period, boys are taller and heavier than girls. Girls have more subcutaneous fat than boys at all ages and the differences become greater with increasing age.

For the health-related fitness components, the sex differences are rather small between 6 and 12 years of age. From the onset of the adolescent growth spurt for boys, the sex differences become especially apparent with girls showing generally no more improvement of their fitness while in boys it still increases. In contrast with cardiorespiratory endurance and the muscular endurance tests, girls perform better than boys for flexibility.

For performance-related fitness tests such as static strength, explosive strength and running speed, boys obtained better results than girls at all ages. The growth curves were parallel between 6 and 12 years of age. From that age onwards, the differences become greater. For the flamingo balance test and for plate tapping, no substantial sex differences were noted.

Sexual dimorphism in motor fitness components can be explained by a large number of factors, such as differences in physiological, biochemical and endocrinological characteristics which undoubtedly influence physical fitness. Body size and body composition are important factors that affect performance in a number of health-related and motor fitness tests. Body size and subcutaneous fatness have no or little effect on flexibility, speed of limb movement and balance, but for cardiorespiratory endurance, the different strength tests and for running speed, they play a significant role in the explanation of the observed sex differences. However, when sex differences are controlled for subcutaneous fatness, weight and height, boys perform still significantly better during adolescence in all strength tests as well as regarding cardiorespiratory endurance. Therefore, other factors such as social and motivational variables, sex differences in physical activity and role patterns may contribute to the explanation of sex differences in physical fitness.

Acknowledgments

This study was supported by BLOSO, the Administration of Physical Education, Sport and Open Air Activities.

References

1. Malina RM, Bouchard C: Growth, Maturation, and Physical Activity. Champaign, Human Kinetics, 1991, p 501.
2. Thomas JR, French KE: Gender differences across age in motor performance: A meta-analysis. Psychol Bull 1985;98:260–282.
3. Council of Europe: Handbook for the EUROFIT Tests of Physical Fitness. Strasbourg, Council of Europe Publishing and Documentation Service, 1993.
4. Lefevre J, Beunen G, Borms J, Renson R, Vrijens J, Claessens AL, Van der Aerschot H: EUROFIT testbatterij: leidraad bij de testafneming en referentiewaarden (Bloso jeugdsportcampagne 92–93). Brussel, Bloso, 1993.
5. Lefevre J, Beunen G, Borms J, Vrijens J, Claessens AL, Van der Aerschot H: EUROFIT testbatterij: leidraad bij de testafneming; referentiewaarden voor 6- tot en met 12-jarige jongens en meisjes in Vlaanderen; groeicurven voor 6- tot en met 18-jarige jongens en meisjes in Vlaanderen. Monografie voor lichamelijke opvoeding 22; reeks sportwetenschappen 2. Sint-Amandsberg/Gent, Publicatiefonds voor lichamelijke opvoeding vzw, 1993.
6. Beunen G, Malina RM: Growth and physical performance relative to the timing of the adolescent spurt; in Pandolf KB (ed): Exercise and Sport Sciences Reviews. New York, Macmillan, 1988, pp 503–540.
7. Renson R, Vanreusel B: Physical activity: Movement activities and sport participation; in Simons J, Beunen GP, Renson R, Claessens ALM, Vanreusel B, Lefevre JAV (eds): Growth and Fitness of Flemish Girls. The Leuven Growth Study. HKP Sport Science Monograph Series 3. Champaign, Human Kinetic Books, 1990, pp 151–160.
8. Malina RM: Menarche in athletes: A synthesis and hypothesis. Ann Hum Biol 1983;10:1–24.

Prof. Dr. J. Lefevre, Centre for Physical Development Research, Department of Kinesiology,
Faculty of Physical Education and Physiotherapy, KU Leuven, Tervuursevest 101,
B–3001 Leuven (Belgium)
Tel. +32 16 329084, Fax +32 16 329197
E-Mail johan.lefevre@flok.kuleuven.ac.be

Relationships between Physical Activity, Motor Ability, and Anthropometric Variables in 6-Year-old Estonian Children

Leila Oja, Toivo Jürimäe

Institute of Sport Pedagogy, University of Tartu, Estonia

Introduction

Health-related physical fitness (HRPF) components are associated with important health outcomes and can be modified through physical activity or exercise [1]. The most acceptable components of HRPF include cardiovascular endurance, muscular strength/endurance, flexibility and body composition [1, 2]. These components are included in the most widely used youth fitness testing programs [3, 4].

Studies which have investigated the possible associations between HRPF and physical activity in children have mostly focused on the cardiovascular endurance and body composition components. It is well known that sedentary adults who undergo longitudinal exercise training demonstrate increased cardiovascular endurance [5]. However, the nature of changes with training are less clear in children [6]. As a rule, the association between physical activity and aerobic fitness is only moderate in children [7]. There is also evidence to suggest that adult activity patterns may be established during childhood [8].

Muscular strength, the second important component of HRPF, has been studied less in very young children. The assessment of their muscular strength can be problematic, however, the data obtained from children are consistent despite the testing procedures. Sex-related differences in strength have already been reported as early as 3 years of age [9].

Riddoch and Boreham [10] concluded that the amount and type of physical activity undertaken during preadolescence that is appropriate for health is unknown. On the other hand, appropriate physical activity for children from the viewpoint of behavioral carryover may also have the effect of increasing fitness levels [11]. Unfortunately, television or computer games capture large blocks of children's time, leaving little time for children to be physically active. Most people think that young children are constantly on the move and have boundless energy, however, actual research data indicate the opposite. For example, Sallis et al. [12] reported that children spent 60% of their play time in sedentary activities, such as sitting, standing, talking, and the like, and only 11% in vigorous activities.

Our knowledge about the associations between children's anthropometry, physical fitness and physical activity is insufficient. Thus, the purpose of the present study was to examine the possible relationships between motor ability, physical activity and somatic growth (anthropometry) in a sample of 6-year-old boys and girls.

Materials and methods

In total, 294 6-year-old kindergarten children from Tartu, Estonia were studied (161 boys and 133 girls). The children participated in two physical education lessons per week supervised by a physical education teacher. The parents of the children gave written permission for the testing and confirmed that their child was free from any medical condition that would preclude participation.

The age of the children was expressed in months, height (Martin anthropometer) in centimeters (± 0.1 cm), and body mass (medical balance scale) in kilograms (± 0.05 kg). The body mass index (BMI, kg/m^2) was also calculated. Three series of anthropometric measurements were taken according to the O-scale physique assessment system [13]. The Centurion Kit (Rosscraft, Surrey, Canada) instrumentation was used. In total, eight skinfolds, ten girths and two breadths were measured. All the anthropometric measurements were taken by a single investigator who had completed preliminary training in anthropometry.

The following motor ability tests from the Eurofit [14] test battery were used: Flamingo balance (30 s), handgrip strength of the dominant hand (Lafayette hand dynamometer, USA), sit and reach, plate tapping, standing broad jump, sit-ups, bent arm hang and the 10×5 m shuttle run. The endurance shuttle run test has been validated in our previous research [4] and the 3-min endurance shuttle run was based on the test of Kaneko and Fuchimoto [15]. Two poles (1.5 m high) were placed 10 m apart for the preparation of a straight 10-meter running track along with four points which were marked by tape. The children ran from one side to another, went around the pole, and then returned to the starting point. The distance covered in 3 min was measured (± 5 m). All fitness tests were conducted at the kindergartens in the morning and separate stations were set up for each measurement. There were only 3 or 4 children in the testing area at the same time.

Physical activity was registered using the questionnaire of Harro [24]. This questionnaire has been validated for Estonian children aged 4–8 years. Questionnaires were completed by parents and teachers according to the daily physical activities of the children. Parents reported the duration of several indoor and outdoor activities in minutes during the children's waking hours at home. Another questionnaire was administered by the teacher to assess the mode and duration of various physical activities at the kindergarten.

Means, standard deviations ($\pm$SD) and zero-order correlation coefficients were initially calculated. One-way analysis of variance (ANOVA) and paired t test post hoc procedures were used to examine differences between the sexes. Second-order partial correlations between motor ability tests, physical activity and anthropometry after the statistical removal of age, body height and body mass were also calculated. Stepwise multiple regression analysis was performed with motor ability test results as independent variables and different anthropometric parameters as dependent variables. Significance was set at $p<0.05$.

Results

Mean anthropometric parameters are presented in table 1. In boys, the body height and mass as well as waist girth, and humerus and femur breadths were significantly higher in comparison with girls. All the skinfold thickness results were higher ($p<0.05$) in girls.

Motor ability test results are presented in table 2. Boys had better results in handgrip strength, standing broad jump and endurance shuttle run, while the results in the Flamingo balance test were better in girls. There were no significant between-group differences in other motor ability tests. Girls were more physically active in the indoor activities ($p<0.05$; table 2). There were no other significant differences in other physical activity scores between the sexes.

Second-order partial correlations between anthropometry and motor ability tests after the effects of age, height and mass were statistically removed are presented in table 3. There were only a few significant correlations between anthropometry and motor ability tests. The girths were more related ($p<0.05$) to motor ability test results than skinfolds. The handgrip strength was more related to anthropometric parameters than the other motor ability tests. As a rule, significant second-order partial correlation coefficients were lower in comparison with zero-order correlations.

Second-order partial correlations between motor ability and physical activity after removing the effects of age, height and mass are presented in table 4. In boys, the indoor passive activities influenced the results of endurance shuttle run ($r=0.26$) and outdoor passive activities decreased the results of the bent arm hang ($r=-0.25$). In girls, the outdoor passive activities increased the results of the 10×5 m shuttle run ($r=-0.20$) and plate tapping ($r=-0.21$). Zero-order correlation analysis indicated that there were statistically significant correlations between indoor passive activities and Flamingo balance ($r=-0.24$), standing broad jump ($r=-0.21$) and endurance shuttle run ($r=0.30$), while indoor active activities increased handgrip strength ($r=0.20$) in boys. In addition, outdoor passive activities increased the results of plate tapping ($r=-0.20$) and handgrip strength ($r=0.24$) and decreased the results

Table 1. Anthropometric parameters of kindergarten children (mean ± SD)

	Boys (n = 161)	Girls (n = 133)	p
Age, months	75.3 ± 9.7	75.4 ± 4.4	NS
Height, cm	121.0 ± 5.8	119.6 ± 5.3	<0.05
Weight, kg	22.1 ± 3.0	21.4 ± 2.9	<0.05
BMI	15.1 ± 1.6	15.0 ± 1.4	NS
Skinfolds, mm			
Triceps	7.9 ± 1.7	8.9 ± 2.1	<0.001
Subscapular	4.7 ± 1.2	5.2 ± 1.3	<0.001
Biceps	4.1 ± 1.5	4.7 ± 1.4	<0.001
Suprailiac	4.2 ± 2.0	5.0 ± 2.0	<0.001
Supraspinal	3.8 ± 1.3	5.0 ± 1.8	<0.001
Abdominal	5.4 ± 2.5	6.7 ± 3.7	<0.001
Mid-thigh	10.4 ± 3.6	12.7 ± 4.1	<0.001
Medial calf	8.4 ± 2.9	10.1 ± 3.2	<0.001
Girths, cm			
Relaxed arm	17.8 ± 1.5	17.8 ± 1.5	NS
Flexed arm	19.1 ± 1.8	19.0 ± 1.5	NS
Forearm	17.5 ± 1.6	17.2 ± 1.7	NS
Wrist	13.3 ± 1.2	13.1 ± 1.2	NS
Chest	58.1 ± 6.6	57.1 ± 3.5	NS
Waist	54.5 ± 4.0	53.2 ± 3.8	<0.01
Gluteal	61.7 ± 4.7	62.0 ± 4.8	NS
Thigh	33.7 ± 4.5	34.3 ± 3.8	NS
Calf	24.4 ± 1.8	24.5 ± 2.2	NS
Ankle	17.6 ± 1.6	17.4 ± 1.7	NS
Breadths, cm			
Humerus	3.9 ± 0.7	3.7 ± 0.7	<0.05
Femur	6.2 ± 0.8	5.9 ± 0.7	<0.01

NS = Not significant.

of the bent arm hang ($r = -0.30$) in boys. In girls, there were close relationships between indoor passive activities and bent arm hang ($r = 0.25$). Outdoor passive activities increased the results of the 10×5 m shuttle run ($r = -0.24$), plate tapping ($r = -0.26$) and standing broad jump ($r = 0.21$) in girls.

Stepwise multiple regression analysis indicated that only a few anthropometric parameters influenced the results of motor ability tests (table 5). The

Table 2. The mean motor ability tests results and physical activities of different intensities (mean ± SD)

	Boys (n = 161)	Girls (n = 133)	p
Motor ability tests			
Flamingo balance, mistakes	8.0 ± 3.7	5.8 ± 3.3	<0.001
Handgrip strength, kg	9.2 ± 4.5	8.0 ± 5.1	<0.05
Sit and reach, cm	21.2 ± 5.6	21.7 ± 5.9	NS
Plate tapping, s	21.3 ± 4.3	20.5 ± 3.9	NS
Standing broad jump, cm	110.0 ± 15.7	101.0 ± 15.9	<0.001
Sit-ups, n/30 s	12.0 ± 4.4	10.7 ± 3.5	NS
Bent arm hang, s	12.0 ± 10.7	11.7 ± 14.9	NS
10 × 5 m shuttle run, s	23.8 ± 2.2	24.1 ± 2.0	NS
Endurance shuttle run, m	408.0 ± 50.2	388.8 ± 49.8	<0.001
Physical activity			
Indoor activities			
Passive, min/day	490.6 ± 105.7	474.9 ± 129.4	NS
Passive, %/day	70.0	73.8	
Active, min/day	52.9 ± 40.5	64.6 ± 41.8	<0.01
Active, %/day	6.7	6.5	
Outdoor activities			
Passive, min/day	127.3 ± 78.3	133.5 ± 55.4	NS
Passive, %/day	16.6	14.6	
Active, min/day	49.2 ± 37.5	47.0 ± 31.8	NS
Active, %/day	6.7	5.1	

NS = Not significant.

girths predominated in different models in comparison with skinfolds and breadths. The results of handgrip strength were more dependent on the anthropometry than the other motor ability test results ($R^2 = 31.54$ in boys and $R^2 = 26.89$ in girls).

Discussion

6-year-old Estonian children were slightly taller and had relatively lower body mass and BMI in comparison with 6- to 7-year-old Czech children [16, 17]. Recent investigations have confirmed that the mean height of Estonian children is higher and the body mass is similar to 'European children' of 6.5

Table 3. Second-order partial correlations between anthropometry and motor ability after the effects of age, height and weight removed

	Flamingo balance		Handgrip strength		Sit and reach		Standing broad jump		10 × 5 m shuttle run		Sit-ups		Bent arm hang		Plate tapping		Endurance shuttle run	
	boys	girls	boys	girls	boys	girls	boys	girls	boys	girls	boys	girls	boys	girls	boys	girls	boys	girls
Skinfolds																		
Triceps	−0.05	0.02	−0.03	−0.04	0.09	0.05	−0.02	−0.20*	−0.03	0.03	−0.03	−0.09	−0.07	0.05	−0.02	0.06	0.03	−0.02
Subscapular	0.04	0.11	0.07	−0.02	0.09	−0.04	0.02	−0.00	−0.00	−0.01	−0.04	−0.07	−0.11	−0.00	0.07	−0.11	−0.03	0.10
Biceps	0.03	−0.03	−0.02	−0.16	0.01	−0.19	−0.07	0.07	0.04	−0.05	−0.01	−0.07	−0.05	−0.11	0.01	−0.05	−0.07	−0.08
Suprailiac	−0.01	0.12	0.16	0.18	0.01	0.10	−0.14	0.02	0.02	0.12	−0.05	0.01	−0.18	−0.07	0.05	0.02	0.01	0.03
Supraspinal	−0.11	0.17	−0.27**	−0.15	−0.09	0.04	0.18	−0.04	−0.09	−0.22*	−0.07	−0.17	−0.04	−0.05	0.10	0.16	−0.11	−0.07
Abdominal	0.01	−0.07	0.01	0.07	0.00	−0.10	−0.11	0.07	−0.01	−0.03	−0.02	0.13	−0.13	0.03	0.01	0.06	−0.08	−0.01
Mid-thigh	0.00	−0.04	−0.09	−0.20*	−0.03	0.09	0.00	−0.03	0.03	0.04	−0.07	0.05	0.01	0.01	0.03	−0.03	−0.08	−0.09
Medial calf	0.23*	0.11	0.11	−0.13	0.02	0.04	0.02	−0.14	0.07	0.17	−0.08	0.12	0.00	0.02	0.12	−0.03	0.02	−0.12
Girths																		
Relaxed arm	−0.02	−0.01	−0.16	0.09	0.19	−0.01	−0.05	−0.12	−0.06	0.10	0.04	0.00	−0.11	0.02	0.01	−0.07	0.15	−0.11
Flexed arm	−0.01	−0.01	0.18	−0.07	−0.14	0.13	0.01	0.13	−0.08	−0.04	0.04	0.05	−0.08	−0.00	0.00	0.03	0.10	0.18
Forearm	0.11	0.09	0.32**	0.31**	−0.08	0.02	0.08	0.00	−0.02	0.09	0.11	0.00	−0.24*	0.03	−0.05	0.08	0.21*	0.09
Wrist	−0.00	−0.02	−0.10	−0.11	0.03	−0.08	−0.10	0.05	−0.00	0.03	−0.00	−0.02	−0.12	−0.02	−0.08	−0.05	0.20*	0.06
Chest	−0.11	−0.03	−0.01	0.05	−0.22*	−0.13	0.22*	0.11	−0.21*	−0.10	−0.05	−0.08	0.00	−0.08	0.02	−0.14	0.09	−0.11
Waist	−0.04	0.11	−0.02	0.15	0.02	−0.01	0.02	0.05	−0.01	0.05	0.07	0.00	−0.15	0.07	0.02	0.02	0.26**	0.11
Gluteal	0.01	−0.08	−0.08	−0.18	0.04	−0.16	0.09	0.14	−0.14	−0.14	0.01	−0.17	−0.08	−0.08	0.08	0.02	0.13	−0.02
Thigh	0.06	0.02	0.24*	0.07	−0.11	0.06	0.11	0.18	−0.07	0.12	0.12	0.17	−0.18	0.02	−0.00	−0.20*	0.10	0.03
Calf	−0.02	0.10	−0.05	−0.16	−0.05	0.02	−0.01	−0.14	−0.04	−0.19	0.09	−0.07	−0.11	0.03	−0.01	0.00	0.07	0.04
Ankle	0.00	−0.02	0.04	0.02	0.10	0.03	0.00	0.11	−0.04	0.04	0.01	0.10	−0.04	0.01	−0.04	−0.21*	0.11	−0.10
Breadths																		
Humerus	0.01	0.14	0.04	0.26**	0.03	0.04	−0.10	−0.15	−0.01	0.17	0.04	−0.02	−0.10	0.03	−0.01	0.07	0.10	0.10
Femur	0.02	−0.03	0.35**	0.13	0.14	0.08	−0.06	−0.02	0.04	−0.04	0.03	−0.07	−0.11	−0.08	−0.07	0.24*	0.20*	0.04

*p<0.05; **p<0.01.

Table 4. Second-order partial correlations between motor ability and physical activity after the effects of age, height and weight removed

	Indoor passive activities		Indoor active activities		Outdoor passive activities		Outdoor active activities	
	boys	girls	boys	girls	boys	girls	boys	girls
Flamingo balance	–0.15	0.08	0.01	–0.05	–0.01	0.16	0.00	–0.04
Handgrip strength	–0.13	0.09	0.09	0.11	–0.04	–0.04	0.05	–0.19
Sit and reach	0.00	0.06	0.11	0.03	0.04	–0.03	0.13	0.03
Plate tapping	–0.04	–0.00	–0.03	0.03	–0.07	0.05	0.00	–0.21*
Standing broad jump	–0.05	0.05	–0.05	0.05	0.03	–0.06	–0.13	0.07
Sit-ups	–0.19	0.19	–0.05	0.07	0.12	–0.08	–0.11	0.01
Bent arm hang	0.05	0.05	–0.02	–0.09	–0.25**	0.07	0.15	–0.05
10 × 5 m shuttle run	0.02	0.14	0.19	0.04	–0.05	–0.20*	0.08	–0.16
Endurance shuttle run	0.26**	0.16	–0.01	0.05	–0.03	0.10	–0.08	–0.02

*p < 0.05; **p < 0.01.

years of age [18]. Similar to other investigations [17], sex differences were identified in skinfold thicknesses, that is, in girls, all the measured skinfold thicknesses were thicker in comparison with boys (table 1). The better height and mass parameters in Estonian children could be explained by the 1- to 2-year participation in regular physical education lessons. Previous research has indicated that children participating in the compulsory physical education programs are taller and their body mass is higher [16].

Play (both inside and outside) is the most natural way for kindergarten children to be active [19] but watching television is a potential distraction [20]. In the current study, girls were significantly more active than boys in indoor activities (table 2). However, Gilliam et al. [21] suggested that the duration of activities at a heart rate of 101–120 beats·min^{-1} was longer in 6- to 7-year-old girls than in boys. In contrast, Durant et al. [22] concluded that activities at heart rate > 120 beats·min^{-1} were slightly longer in 5- to 7-year-old girls than in boys.

Our understanding of the factors that may affect physical activity and the physical fitness level in children could be relevant to the modification of physical activity in childhood. It has been suggested that the physical activity and physical fitness of Estonian children are relatively poor [23, 24]. In the present study, once the influence of age, body height and body mass were excluded there were few relationships between physical fitness and physical activity. Results in the present study contradict results of studies of other 9-

Table 5. Stepwise multiple regression analysis summary between motor ability test results (independent variables) and anthropometry (dependent variables)

	Boys				Girls			
	dependent variables	R^2	F	p	dependent variables	R^2	F	p
Flamingo balance	Age Calf girth Flexed arm girth	16.31	2.87	<0.01	Supraspinal skinfold	4.90	1.02	<0.01
Handgrip strength	Supraspinal skinfold Relaxed arm girth Thigh girth Femur breadths	31.54	3.56	<0.001	Height Biceps skinfold Waist girth Humerus breadths	26.89	2.66	<0.001
Sit and reach	BMI	5.13	1.23	<0.05	Height Thigh girth	8.55	1.00	<0.01
Plate tapping					Forearm girth Supraspinal skinfold Ankle girth Femur breadths	15.41	2.51	<0.001
Standing broad jump	Chest girths	6.29	1.69	<0.05	Triceps skinfold	6.41	1.02	<0.01
Sit-ups	Forearm girths BMI	5.27	0.98	<0.05				
Bent arm hang	Forearm girths	3.82	0.77	<0.05				
10 × 5 m shuttle run	Chest girths Thigh girths Calf girths	9.24	3.00	<0.01	Age Calf girths Humerus breadths	15.25	3.04	<0.001
Endurance shuttle run	Gluteal girths Femur breadths	11.11	2.96	<0.001				

R^2 = Coefficient of determination × 100.

year-old children where some association was reported between physical activity and aerobic fitness [25]. Sunnegardh and Bratteby [26] reported a significant relationship between maximal O_2 consumption (VO_{2max}) and the level of physical activity in 8-year-old boys but not in girls of the same age. Disparity in the results may be accounted for by the methodology employed to measure physical activity [27] and also the unquantified genetic component [28].

For boys, the endurance shuttle run test results correlated significantly with indoor passive activities (see table 4). Daily activities of moderate to high intensity have been shown to correlate with VO_{2max} [7] and the relationships between VO_{2max} and daily physical activity have been reported to be nonsignificant in slightly older boys [29].

There were only weak significant second order partial correlations between anthropometry and motor ability tests in 6-year-old children. Skinfold thicknesses did not influence the results of the endurance shuttle run in boys or girls (table 3), whilst girths (forearm, wrist, waist) were more important in boys. Stepwise multiple regression analysis indicated that gluteal girth and femur breadth accounted for about 11% of the variance in endurance shuttle run performance (table 5). These results were surprising as the body fat percentage has been reported to decrease the results of the endurance shuttle run test in older children [30]. Pařízková et al. [16] indicated that the characteristics of the economy of work of the cardiorespiratory system correlated positively with circumferential and breadth measurements in preschool children. In the present study, only forearm, wrist and waist girths, and femur breadths correlated significantly with endurance shuttle run test results using second-order partial correlations in boys (table 3).

Mean results of handgrip strength (table 2) were slightly lower than in children of the same age in the USA [31] with significantly better results in boys than in girls. The mean results for Estonian girls were moderately better than in Flemish girls of the same age [32]. Consistent with Jones and Mills [33] the researchers believe that the strength tests used were suitable for use with young children. Close relationships have been reported between body height and mass, and isometric strength characteristics in older (9- to 18-year-old) children [34]. After removing the influence of age, height and mass only a few anthropometric parameters influenced the results of handgrip strength in the children tested (table 3).

An earlier study [35] has reported on the inability of 4- to 6-year-olds to maintain balance. However, there were no difficulties in using the well-known Flamingo balance test in the present study, except that the testing time was decreased to 30 s because of fatigue of the children's leg muscles. Balance is a very specific motor ability and the results of the balance test do not depend on the anthropometric parameters or physical activity (tables 3, 4).

Summary and Conclusions

The purpose of the present study was to examine the possible relationships between motor ability, physical activity and somatic growth in a sample of 6-year-old Estonian boys and girls. Anthropometric measurements were taken according to the O-scale physique assessment system. The following motor ability tests were used from the Eurofit test battery: Flamingo balance (30 s), handgrip strength, sit and reach, plate tapping, standing broad jump, sit-ups, bent arm hang and 10×5 m shuttle run. A 3-min endurance shuttle run was also used. Physical activity was registered using the questionnaire of Harro [24]. In boys, body height and mass as well as waist girth and humerus and femur breadths were significantly higher in comparison with girls. All skinfold thicknesses were thicker ($p < 0.05$) in girls. Handgrip strength, standing broad jump and endurance shuttle run test results were better ($p < 0.05$) in boys. Flamingo balance results were better in girls, and girls were more active in indoor tasks. There were only a few significant correlations between anthropometry and motor ability tests using second-order partial correlations when age, height and mass were statistically removed. As a rule, only one or two physical activity components significantly influenced motor ability tests results. Stepwise multiple regression analysis indicated that girths predominated more in models different than skinfolds or breadths. The results of handgrip strength were more dependent on the anthropometry than other motor ability tests ($R^2 = 31.54$ in boys and $R^2 = 26.89$ in girls). Results indicate that motor ability does not depend on the amount of physical activity and anthropometric variables in 6-year-old boys and girls.

References

1. Pate RR, Shephard RJ: Characteristics of physical fitness in youth; in Gisolfi C, Lamb D (eds): Perspectives in Exercise Science and Sports Medicine: Youth, Exercise, and Sport. Indianapolis, Benchmark Press, 1989, vol 2, pp 1–46.
2. Caspersen CJ, Powell KE, Christenson GM: Physical activity, exercise, and physical fitness: Definitions and distinctions for health-related research. Public Health Rep 1985;100:126–131.
3. Fitnessgram User's Manual. Dallas, Institute for Aerobic Research, 1988.
4. Oja L, Jürimäe T: Assessment of motor ability in 4- and 5-year-old children. Am J Hum Biol 1997; 9:659–664.
5. Haskell WL, Leon AS, Caspersen CJ: Cardiovascular benefits and assessment of physical activity and physical fitness in adults. Med Sci Sports Exerc 1992;24(suppl):S210-S220.
6. Sady SP: Cardiorespiratory exercise training in children. Clin Sports Med 1986;5:493–514.
7. Pate RR, Dowda M, Ross JG: Associations between physical fitness in American children. Am J Dis Child 1990;14:1123–1129.
8. Armstrong N: Children's cardiopulmonary fitness and physical activity patterns: The European scene; in Blimkie CJR, Bar-Or O (eds): New Horizons in Pediatric Exercise Science. Champaign, Human Kinetics, 1995, pp 181–193.
9. Armstrong N, Welsman J: Young People and Physical Activity. London, Oxford University Press, 1997.
10. Riddoch CJ, Boreham CAG: The health-related physical activity of children. Sports Med 1995;29: 86–102.
11. Sallis JF: A commentary on children and fitness: A public health perspective. Res Q Exerc Sport 1987;58:326–330.
12. Sallis JF, Patterson RL, McKenzie TL, Nader PR: Family variables and physical activity in preschool children. J Dev Behav Pediatr 1988;9:57–61.

13   Ward R, Ross WD, Leyland AJ, Selbie S: The Advanced O-Scale Physique Assessment System. Burnaby, Kinemetrix, 1989.
14   Eurofit: European Test of Physical Fitness. Rome, Council of Europe, Committee for the Development of Sport, 1988.
15   Kaneko M, Fuchimoto T: Endurance performance capacity of 7 to 18 year old boys and girls assessed by the 'shuttle stamina test'; in Claessens AL, Lefevre J, van den Eynde B (eds): World-Wide Variation in Physical Fitness. Leuven, Institute of Physical Education, 1993, pp 80–86.
16   Pařízková J, Adamec A, Berdychová J, Čermák J, Horná J, Teplý Z: Growth, Fitness and Nutrition in Preschool Children. Prague, Charles University, 1984.
17   Pařízková J: Nutrition, Physical Activity, and Health in Early Life. Boca Raton, CRC Press, 1996.
18   Nutrient and Energy Intakes for the European Community: Report of the Scientific Committee for Food. Luxemburg, Directorate-General, Industry, Office for Official Publications, 1993, ser 31.
19   Rippe JM, Weissberg RP, Seefeldt V: The purpose of play: A framework for improving childhood health and psychological and physical development. Med Exerc Nutr Health 1993;2:225–231.
20   Åstrand P-O: Physical activity and fitness: Evolutionary perspective and trends for the future; in Bouchard C, Shephard RJ, Stephens T (eds): Physical Activity, Fitness, and Health. Champaign, Human Kinetics, 1994, pp 98–105.
21   Gilliam TB, Freedson PS, Geenen DL: Physical activity patterns determined by heart rate monitoring in 6–7-year-old children. Med Sci Sports Exerc 1981;13:65–67.
22   Durant RH, Baranovski T, Davis H: Reliability and variability of indicators of heart-rate monitoring in children. Med Sci Sports Exerc 1993;25:389–395.
23   Raudsepp L, Jürimäe T: Physical activity, fitness, and adiposity of prepubertal girls. Pediatr Exerc Sci 1996;8:259–267.
24   Harro M: Validation of a questionnaire to assess physical activity of children ages 4–8 years. Res Q Exerc Sport 1997;68:259–268.
25   Kikuchi S, Rona RJ, Chinn S: Physical fitness of 9 year olds in England: Related factors. J Epidemiol Community Health 1995;49:180–185.
26   Sunnegardh J, Bratteby LE: Maximal oxygen uptake, anthropometry and physical activity in a randomly selected sample of 8- and 13-year-old children in Sweden. Eur J Appl Physiol 1987;56:266–272.
27   Caspersen CJ: Physical activity epidemiology: Concepts, methods, and applications to exercise science; in Pandolf K (ed): Exercise and Sport Sciences Reviews. Baltimore, Williams & Wilkins, 1989, vol 17, pp 423–473.
28   Bouchard C, Lortie G: Heredity and endurance performance. Sports Med 1984;1:38–64.
29   Cunningham D, Paterson D, Blimkie C, Donner A: Development of cardiorespiratory function in circumpubertal boys: A longitudinal study. J Appl Physiol 1985;56:301–307.
30   Slaughter MH, Lohman TG, Misner JE: Association of somatotype and body composition to physical performance in 7–12-year-old girls. J Sports Med 1980;20:189–198.
31   Malina RM, Bouchard C: Growth, Maturation and Physical Activity. Champaign, Human Kinetics, 1991, pp 115–131.
32   Beunen GP, Simons J: Physical growth, maturation and performance; in Simons J, Beunen GP, Renson R, Claessens ALM, van Reusel B, Lefevre JAV (eds): Growth and Fitness of Flemish Girls: The Leuven Growth Study. Champaign, Human Kinetics, 1990, pp 69–118.
33   Jones PA, Mills ME: Muscle strength and training in children; in Mafulli N (ed): Color Atlas of Sports Medicine in Childhood and Adolescence. London, Mosby-Wolfe, pp 101–108.
34   Blimkie CJR: Age and sex associated variation in strength during childhood; in Gisolfi CV, Lamb DR (eds): Perspectives in Exercise Science and Sports Medicine. Indianapolis, Benchmark Press, 1989, vol 2: Youth, Exercise, and Sport, pp 99–161.
35   Shumway-Cook A, Woollacott MH: The growth of stability: Postural from a developmental perspective. J Motor Behav 1985;17:131–147.

Prof. T. Jürimäe, Institute of Sport Pedagogy, Faculty of Exercise and Sport Sciences, University of Tartu, 18 Ülikooli Street, EE2400 Tartu (Estonia)

Aerobic and Anaerobic Performances in Relation to Marginal Malnutrition and Altitude in Bolivian Boys and Girls

Nicole Fellmann, Mario Bedu, Jean Coudert

Laboratory of Physiology and Sports Biology, Faculty of Medicine, Clermont-Ferrand, France

Introduction

Most Bolivian people live at high altitude (HA) in the Andean Altiplano which is the least economically developed region of the country. Numerous studies have reported that the growth in height and weight of highland children is delayed compared to counterparts at sea level. The smaller stature of those living at HA appears to be due to a smaller size at birth and a slower growth period.

It has been concluded that growth retardation at HA is principally the result of the hypoxic environment [1]. However, the prevalence of protein malnutrition in Bolivian children must be taken into account before definitive conclusions can be made. Bolivia is in fact considered to be at middle level of development. In common with other Latin-American countries, Bolivian children who live in poor socioeconomic and hygienic conditions are often exposed to nutritional deprivation. Estimates from de Onis et al. [2] indicate that Latin-American children suffer from marginal nutrition, 20% have low weight for age and 12% low height for age. As a consequence, when children with the same nutritional and socioeconomic status are compared, the physical growth pattern of Andean HA children is similar to their respective peers living at low altitude (LA), providing evidence of the predominance of nutritional effects on growth retardation at HA [see references cited in 1 and 3].

Decreased spontaneous activity and a reduced body size as an adaptation to marginal malnutrition have negative effects on physical fitness and performance of children living under poor nutrition conditions. Consequently, in order to separate the effect of hypoxia from malnutrition on physical performances, children must be matched for altitude levels and also for socioeconomic and nutritional status.

Until now, few studies have focused on the performance of Bolivian children in relation to malnutrition and altitude. The first papers from Greksa and his collaborators [4–6] gave information on maximal oxygen consumption in children of different genetic and socioeconomic backgrounds. More recently, our laboratory, in collaboration with members of the Instituto Boliviano de Biologia de Altura (IBBA) in La Paz, has thoroughly investigated performances requiring energy from aerobic and anaerobic metabolism, using various laboratory and field tests in circumpubertal boys and girls of high (HSES) and low (LSES) socioeconomic status living at HA and LA. These results will be described in this paper.

Methods, Results and Discussion

Subjects

Since 1982, 287 boys and 151 girls aged 7–15 years have been studied in Bolivia. The investigations were carried out at HA in La Paz (altitude 3,600 m, mean barometric pressure 500 mm Hg and ambient temperature 16 °C) and at LA in Santa Cruz de la Sierra [altitude 420 m, mean barometric pressure 725 mm Hg and ambient temperature: 21 °C (winter season)]. Children were either natives or had lived for 3 years or more at HA or at LA.

HA environment not only results in hypoxic stress but also in cold and in hypobaric exposure. However, chronic exposure to an altitude of 3,600 m does not induce the same adaptive responses as those seen in mountaineers during climbing expeditions at higher altitude. In these transitory situations, additional factors such as intense cold, appetite loss, confining, low spontaneous activities with a decrease in muscle and fat mass worsen the more severe hypoxia. These changes are never observed in the Andean highland population living at the altitude of La Paz. Conversely, the very hot and humid climate during summer in the tropical zone of Santa Cruz may have a negative effect on physical performance in addition to the nutrition impact.

Socioeconomic Levels

In the past 30 years, La Paz and Santa Cruz have undergone a rapid growth due to an influx of population from rural areas. The result has been the development of underprivileged areas which have sprung up in successive layers around the periphery of each city. The reduced socioeconomic and hygienic conditions of these areas have resulted in a high incidence of undernutrition among the children. Girls and boys were judged to belong to the lower or upper socioeconomic level by their place of residence and the type of school they attend (private for HSES and public for LSES). The level of socioeconomic status was assessed by using a questionnaire during a home visit at which their parents were present.

Marginal malnutrition is only one aspect of the reality of a low socioeconomic status which is often associated with poor hygienic conditions. This leads to a high incidence of infectious diseases and intestinal parasitosis which induce malabsorption of food and worsen the poor nutrient intake. Additionally, social and cultural factors make it difficult to isolate the effect of actual malnutrition on stunted growth and lower physical performance.

Ethnic background in South America is also often associated with socioeconomic status. Children from middle and upper-class families appear to be predominantly of European ancestry, while children of poor socioeconomic status have both Spanish and Ameridian (Aymaras, Quetchuas) ancestry. However, due to considerable interbreeding, it is often very difficult to be definitive regarding their genetic background. Consequently, the lack of distinct groups with similar ancestry does not enable one to distinguish the role of genetic factors from environmental effects.

Nutritional Status

In the current study, nutritional status was evaluated by anthropometric and biological parameters. Dietary information and daily physical activity data indicate the following. (1) Altitude has no effect on the physical growth and the nutritional intake [1, 3, 7, 8]. The stature and weight of HSES boys and girls at HA are within the normal range for well-nourished children of the same age living at LA (fig. 1, 2). Moreover, in HSES children the energy and nutrient intakes which are higher than recommended are similar at HA and LA. (2) In LSES groups, low weight for age and low height for age but normal weight for height give evidence of a long-term marginal malnutrition which has been shown to occur during early childhood [1, 7, 8]. At HA and at LA, their physical growth is delayed by approximately 9 months to 2 years, compared to their HSES counterparts according to gender. This is more pronounced in boys (fig. 1, 2). A reduced muscle mass and a normal fat mass when compared to American children confirm the marginal malnutrition.

In addition, the measurements of biological markers, the nutritional screening and activity interview indicate a tendency towards a current malnutrition in LSES groups. Although protein intake (total and per kilogram body weight) shows no deficiencies in both LSES groups, there is a large difference in quality. The protein intake of LSES children is mainly of vegetable origin, whereas HSES children consume adequate animal products to have high quality protein. Moreover protein and fat intakes are significantly lower in LSES groups with an energy

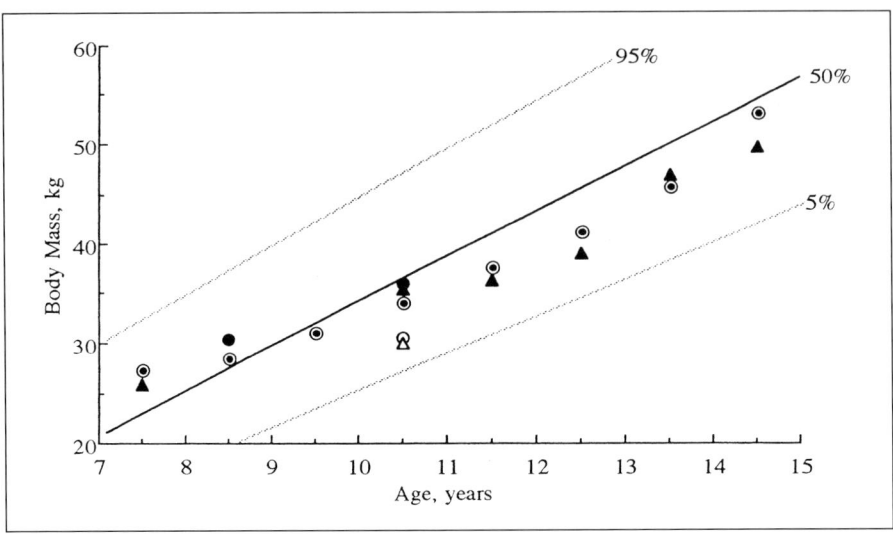

Fig. 1. Changes in body mass between the age of 7 and 15 years in boys of upper socioeconomic class living at HA in La Paz (▲) and at LA in Clermont-Ferrand (France; ☉) or Santa Cruz (●), and in boys from low socioeconomic background living at HA (△) and in Santa Cruz (○) [from 8, 12, 14, 18, 20, 22]. Solid (50th) and dotted (5th and 95th) lines represent percentiles of the US reference.

contribution of 13–17 versus 23–27% for fat and 11 versus 16% for proteins [3]. At LA in LSES groups, the higher frequency of intestinal parasitosis than in HSES ones (97 vs. 58%) [7] and a higher physical activity (household task involvement; +30%) weaken the precarious equilibrium between energy intake and expenditure [3, 9]. Finally, plasma prealbumin (–16%) [8] and insulin-like growth factor (IgFI) concentrations (–19%) [10] which are lower in LSES groups but within the normal range give evidence in some cases of current marginal malnutrition in the poor socioeconomic groups.

As a consequence, these two environmental factors (altitude and socioeconomic and nutritional conditions) will modulate physical performance of the children living in Bolivia. An extension of this work was comparing Bolivian children with their French counterparts living in Clermont-Ferrand (altitude 330 m, n = 191) who were judged to be well-nourished.

Aerobic Performance

Aerobic metabolism was evaluated by direct mesurement of $\dot{V}O_{2max}$ and by a field test (20-meter shuttle run).

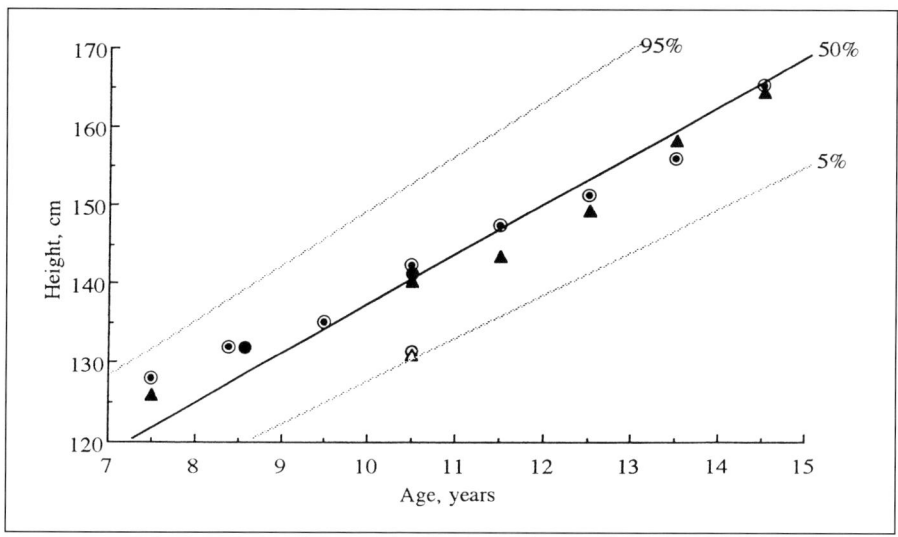

Fig. 2. Changes in height between the age of 7 and 15 years in boys of upper socioeconomic class living at HA in La Paz (▲) and at LA in Clermont-Ferrand (France; ⊙) or Santa Cruz (●), and in boys from low socioeconomic background living at HA (△) and in Santa Cruz (○) [from 8, 12, 14, 18, 20, 22]. Solid (50th) and dotted (5th and 95th) lines represent percentiles of the US reference.

Effect of Altitude

As in adults [11], aerobic performance at the altitude of La Paz is reduced in HSES as well as in LSES children (fig. 3). The decrease varies from 8 to 22% according to the age, sex, the level of physical activity, the groups compared, the methodology used and how the results were expressed (in absolute terms or related to body weight or muscle mass). The performance evaluated from the shuttle running strengthens the laboratory results. The maximal aerobic velocity is also lower at HA (–9%) on pubertal and prepubertal boys as compared to French children of the same age [12].

The smaller difference observed between children from La Paz and Santa Cruz (8%) than La Paz and Clermont-Ferrand (15–22%) may be due to the very poor level of physical fitness of LA boys [8] and girls [7] (fig. 3). As mentioned above, Santa Cruz is located in a tropical zone and has a very hot and humid climate for 9 months of the year. These ambient conditions and also sociocultural factors may lead to reduced voluntary physical activity among these children. In effect, the activity profile shows that girls at LA are less active than their peers at HA (–26%) [3] and could partly explain their very poor VO_{2max}, below the values usually obtained at LA.

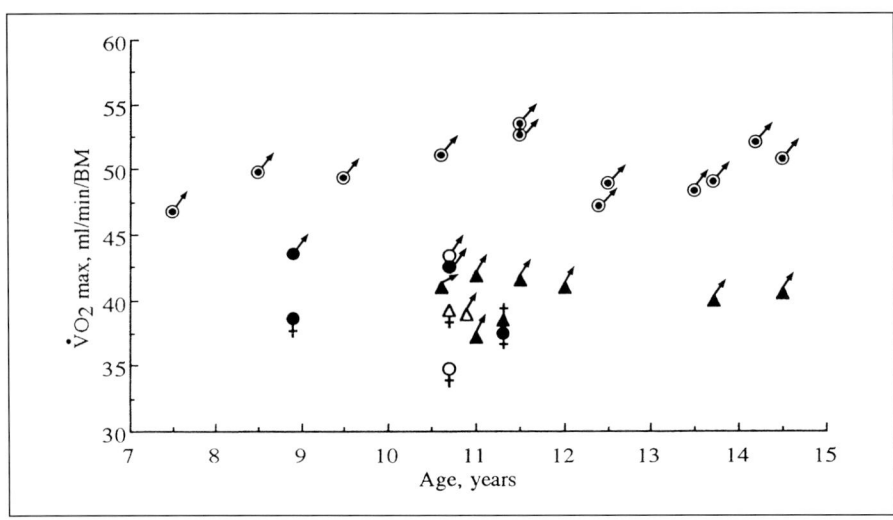

Fig. 3. Maximal oxygen consumption ($\dot{V}O_{2max}$) from the age of 7 and 15 years living at HA in La Paz from high (▲) and low (△) socioeconomic background, and in lowland children from upper socioeconomic class living in Santa Cruz (●) or in Clermont-Ferrand (☉) and from low socio-economic background living in Santa Cruz (○). Arrows represent boys, crosses girls [from 7, 8, 12, 14, 18, 20, 22]. BM = Body mass.

At HA, the values are of the same order of magnitude as found by Greksa et al. [4, 6] in 9- to 13-year-old boys from high and low class families (40–46 ml/min/kg) and by Andersen [13] in 10- to 12-year-old Ethiopian boys living at the altitude of 3,000 m (40 ml/min/kg). Moreover, in contrast to Frisancho's hypothesis on adults, Greksa and Haas [4] demonstrated that the length of residence at HA during childhood does not alter maximal work performance. $\dot{V}O_{2max}$ did not differ significantly between boys (aged 8.8–13.1 years) born at HA (39.6 ml/min/kg) and boys born at LA who migrated to La Paz between the age of 6–11 years (40.2 ml/min/kg).

With training, $\dot{V}O_{2max}$ can reach higher values. Greksa et al. [5] found in trained swimmers residing in La Paz, 52 ml/min/kg for a 15-year-old boy and 47 ml/min/kg for a 13-year-old girl. However, $\dot{V}O_{2max}$ always remained lower (10–20%) in HA swimmers than in selected samples of sea level competitive swimmers.

The limiting factors for $\dot{V}O_{2max}$ at HA are not clearly defined. Although maximal heart rate (HR_{max}) measured during the 20-meter shuttle run is higher than that recorded in the laboratory at the end of maximal exercise [12], HR_{max} at HA is always reduced by 6–15 beats/min according to studies that may induce a lower $\dot{V}O_{2max}$ at HA. From adults' data, the decrease in O_2 pressure gradient between capillaries and mitochondria (linked to the PaO_2 reduction) would also be involved.

Socioeconomic and Nutritional Effect

In liters per minute, $\dot{V}O_{2max}$ of well-nourished children is significantly higher than that of marginally undernourished ones [7, 8]. This decrease is related to their reduced body size because, when corrected for fat-free mass or muscle leg volume or body weight, the difference is eliminated (fig. 3). This observation is strengthened by the fact that when children are matched for their body dimension (that is a comparison between 9-year-old HSES and 11-year-old LSES children), they have similar values for absolute $\dot{V}O_{2max}$ in liters per min (fig. 3) [14]. These data are in line with those obtained by other investigators at LA in Colombian boys and girls aged 6–16 years [15]. The same conclusion has been drawn in respect of physical working capacity (PWC 170) in undernourished Indian boys aged 14–17 years [16].

However, when corrected by body weight, $\dot{V}O_{2max}$ obtained in LA children from Santa Cruz are systematically lower than those reported for Colombian [15] or European children (fig. 3). Mean $\dot{V}O_{2max}$ of HSES children is reduced by 8–14% compared to European and well-fed Colombian children, whereas for LSES children the values are reduced by 20–22% compared to nutritionally deprived Colombian children. A low hemoglobin concentration cannot be an explanatory factor because LSES children with anemia (Hb < 11 g/100 ml) are excluded from the studies. Although HSES cases of obesity (body mass index > 21.5) are also excluded, the high body fat mass, especially in girls (25–26%), induces a lower performance when expressed by unit of body weight. As suggested above, the tropical climate of Santa Cruz combined with sociocultural factors could have led to reduced voluntary activity and physical fitness. The higher sensitivity of girls to these factors explains why the relationship between $\dot{V}O_{2max}$ and fat-free mass is similar for HSES and LSES boys but not for girls [14]. In contrast to Colombian girls studied by Spurr and Reina [15], the reduced muscle mass is not the only contributor to the decreased $\dot{V}O_{2max}$ in Bolivian undernourished girls living in Santa Cruz.

Mean HR_{max} of LSES children is significantly reduced by 7 beats/min at LA as compared to HSES boys and girls. It is unlikely that LSES children give up exercise before exhaustion because no significant socioeconomic status effect is found for the other criteria of maximal exercise (respiratory exchange ratio, blood lactate concentration). However Spurr and Reina [15] have not found such a difference among LSES and HSES Colombian children exercising to exhaustion on a treadmill. More severe malnutrition has been shown to induce changes in cardiac function (electrocardiographic alterations, reduced stroke volume and cardiac output proportionally to weight deficit). Nevertheless, since the same decrease in HR_{max} is found at HA (5–6 beats/min) in undernourished boys and girls, the hypothesis that LSES combined with a mild malnutrition could induce lower HR_{max} in children during exercise needs further investigation.

Anaerobic Performances

Anaerobic metabolism was assessed by field tests (30-meter dash and 30-second shuttle run) plus laboratory tests for the measurement of maximal anaerobic power during a force-velocity test and a 30-second Wingate test, oxygen debt in submaximal and supramaximal exercises, blood lactate concentrations [L] during and after maximal and supramaximal tests and ventilatory anaerobic threshold.

Effect of Altitude [17]

Force-Velocity Test. Irrespective of nutritional status, an altitude of 3,600 m does not modify the anaerobic power developed during a force-velocity test (P_{max}) when HA children are compared to their LA counterparts in Santa Cruz [7, 8] or to French HSES children [18] of the same age (fig. 4). Performance using the corresponding field test (mean velocity during a 30-meter dash) is highly correlated to P_{max} and is the same in French as in Bolivian children living in La Paz [12]. These results suggest that, as in adults, stores of ATP and phosphocreatine which are mainly involved in such tests are not affected by chronic hypoxia [17].

Wingate Test (fig. 5). The results obtained during a 30-second Wingate test are controversial and depend on the HSES groups considered for the comparison and their ages. When compared to their French peers of HSES, the mean power (MP) developed during the test is the same at HA and LA for boys aged 7–8 years, and is reduced at HA in boys aged 11–12 years (–19%) and 14–15 years (–23%) [18]. Likewise, the performance evaluated by a 30-second shuttle run is also significantly reduced at HA by 3–4% for two age groups (11 and 14 years) with Clermont-Ferrand as the LA reference [12]. In contrast, the result is different when the control group at LA is Bolivian. Regardless of socioeconomic background, the 11-year-old boys at HA have the same MP as their counterparts living in Santa Cruz [8], whereas the HA girls have higher values [7]. These discrepancies could result in several factors. During the Wingate test, anaerobic glycolysis may account for a large proportion of the work performed. Therefore, the reduced performance at HA in the former studies could be related to a lower lactate production. [L] at the 2nd minute of recovery is in fact consistently lower at HA (see below) [18]. Another

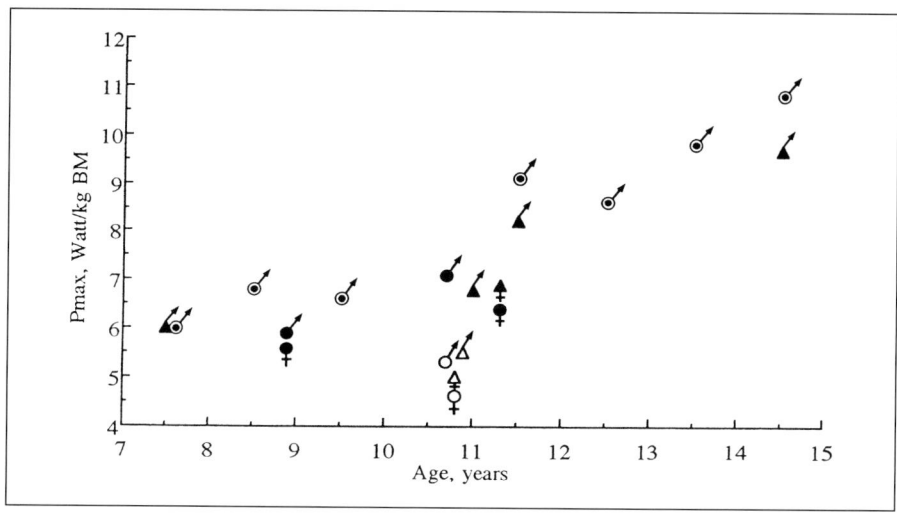

Fig. 4. Changes with age between 7 and 15 years in maximal anaerobic power developed during a force-velocity test (P_{max}) in children living at HA in La Paz from high (▲) and low (△) socioeconomic background, and in lowland children of upper socioeconomic class living in Santa Cruz (●) or in Clermont-Ferrand (☉) and from low socioeconomic background living in Santa Cruz (○). Arrows represent boys, crosses girls [from 7, 8, 14, 18]. BM = Body mass.

possible explanation for a lower MP at HA is a reduced aerobic participation. In effect, since the relative energy contribution of aerobic metabolism during the Wingate test is high, particularly in children, the higher oxygen consumption measured during the whole test at LA (+15 to +24%) may explain the difference in MP [18]. However, we calculated that in order to have exactly the same MP at both altitude by oxygen energy compensation, the mechanical efficiency at HA would theoretically be 42% for the 11-year-old boys and 47% for the group 15 years of age, which is unlikely [17]. This is in line with results obtained in acute hypoxia. When prepubertal children are exposed to acute normoxia at HA and to acute hypoxia at LA, MP is not altered [19]. Finally, the lack of difference between La Paz and Santa Cruz may be due to the poor physical fitness of the children living in Santa Cruz as mentioned above for aerobic performance. MP in HSES Bolivian children is lower than European references at the same age [18] (fig. 5).

The lower MP at HA corresponds to the data obtained in adults [17]. Chronic hypoxia in HA resident adults studied in their home environment (3,700–4,200 m) results in a decrease in MP by 12%. Similarly in untrained students (24 years-old) living in La Paz, MP is reduced by 14% as compared to sedentary French students of the same age [Coudert, unpubl. data].

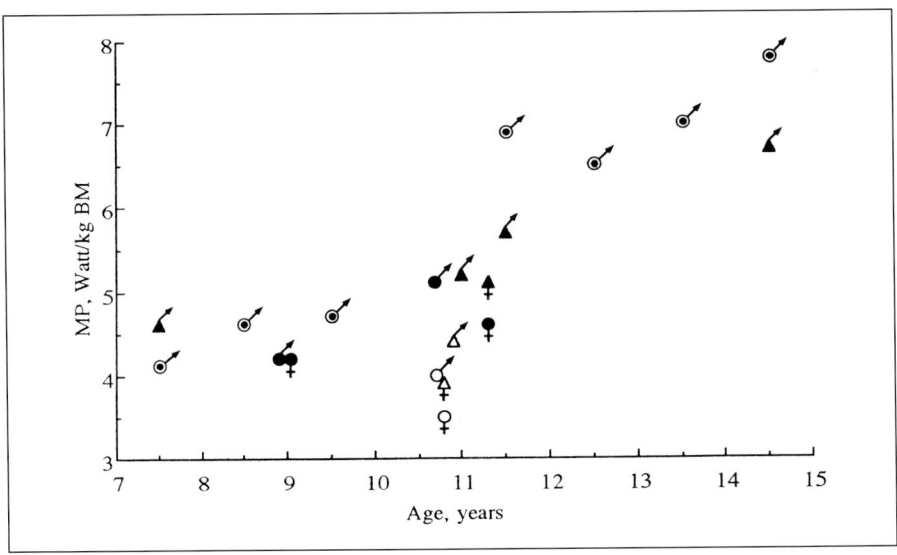

Fig. 5. Mean aerobic power developed during a 30-second Wingate test (MP) in children living at HA in La Paz from high (▲) and low (△) socioeconomic background, and in lowland children from upper socioeconomic class living in Santa Cruz (●) or in Clermont-Ferrand (⊙), and from low socioeconomic background living in Santa Cruz (○). Arrows represent boys, crosses girls [from 7, 8, 14, 18]. BM = Body mass.

Oxygen Debt. When related to percent of $\dot{V}O_{2max}$, O_2 debt during submaximal (20–95% $\dot{V}O_{2max}$) and supramaximal (115% $\dot{V}O_{2max}$) exercises is similar at HA and LA in Clermont-Ferrand from the age of 10–13 years [20]. It is usually admitted that the O_2 corresponding to the slow component of debt is mainly representative of the amount of lactic acid produced at the onset of exercise. Therefore, it can be concluded that HA does not modify the anaerobic capacity in children. These results are in accordance with an equal anaerobic threshold at HA and LA in Clermont-Ferrand using ventilatory and gas exchange indexes (70–75% $\dot{V}O_{2max}$) [20].

Blood Lactate Concentration [17]. The results are inconsistent. [L] measured at the 2nd minute of recovery are either the same at HA as at LA (Clermont-Ferrand or Santa Cruz) after maximal exercise [7, 18, 20] and supramaximal tests [7, 18, 20] or lower at HA as compared to French or Bolivian children after maximal exercises [18], for 30-second Wingate tests [8, 18] and field tests [12]. Even when related to MP which is lower at HA, [L] remains lower than at LA whatever the socioeconomic status [21]. In only one study, [L] is found to be higher at HA after maximal exercise in Bolivian 12-year-old boys than French boys of the same age [22].

These discrepancies could be partly explained by a difference in sexual development. [L] after maximal exercise [22] or a Wingate test [21] are positively correlated with salivary testosterone concentrations ([T]) at HA and LA in French and Bolivian boys. These observations agree with previous reports in humans and animals and give evidence that androgens would have a direct or indirect effect on muscle anaerobic metabolism. At the present time, the mechanism is not clearly understood. Nevertheless, this could explain the higher [L] in 12-year-old boys living in La Paz because of an enhanced anaerobic metabolism linked to an earlier gonadal maturation than in their French counterparts of the same age and of the same HSES [22].

However, in spite of significant correlations between [L] and [T], stepwise regression analyses indicate that [T] is a weak predictor of [L] after the Wingate test (4% of the total explained variance). Therefore, other factors could be involved in lower [L] at HA. Circulating [L] itself does not provide definitive information on muscle lactate production because [L] is a complex function of production, release and removal. On the one hand, the lactate disappearance during the recovery of maximal exercise is faster in HSES boys living in La Paz as compared to their French peers [22]. If the lactate production is not altered by hypoxia, the lower [L] could be the consequence of a more effective lactate removal from blood. On the other hand, numerous studies in adults give evidence of a lower muscle production under chronic hypoxia [17]. Such a finding needs to be verified in children.

Effect of Socioeconomic and Nutritional Status [23]

In contrast to aerobic metabolism, a marginal malnutrition diminishes anaerobic performances of both sexes [7, 8]. P_{max} and MP in absolute terms are reduced in LSES children (by 35–40 and 31–37%, respectively) whatever the altitude at which they lived (3,600 or 420 m). Even when corrected for body mass, lean body mass or muscle leg volume, the anaerobic power remain lower in LSES groups (fig. 4, 5). These differences are more marked in girls [7]. Body dimensions explained only 67% of the variation of the maximal anaerobic power [7]. Therefore apart from quantitative changes (anthropometric characteristics and especially muscle mass) induced by malnutrition, qualitative muscle factors from either psychomotor, biochemical or biomechanical origin could also play a role in the reduced anaerobic power. These conclusions are strengthened when 11-year-old LSES boys and girls are compared to HSES groups who are 2 years younger but have the same anthropometric characteristics as LSES ones: P_{max} and MP remain lower in LSES children [14].

From these data it can be hypothesized that marginal malnutrition during infancy and childhood could have resulted in impaired muscle function [14].

This is supported by numerous studies on structural, metabolic and functional changes occurring in human and animal skeletal muscle as a consequence of malnutrition. Most of these investigations have provided evidence that undernutrition leads to muscular atrophy (reduced fiber diameter and loss of fiber number in some cases). This effect is selective and concerns mainly the fast twitch fibers (FT) whereas the slow twitch fibers (ST) are generally unaffected by malnutrition except for very severe malnutrition. The mechanism underlying the relative sparing of ST in relation to FT fibers is probably dependent on the contractile activity. ST motor units have been shown to be earlier and more frequently recruited than FT ones, resulting in less frequent use and activity of FT fibers. With malnutrition, this relative FT fiber inactivity is amplified because in terms of fuel economy, their metabolism (anaerobic glycolysis) is more costly. This fiber adaptation could be worsened by alterations in the responsiveness of inactive tissue to circulating hormones. Inactive muscle tissue becomes more responsive to catabolic hormones and less responsive to anabolic hormones. Unfortunately, the malnutrition induces a decrease in insulin and IgFI, and an increase in glucocorticoid concentrations. Consequently, inhibition of protein synthesis and enhancement of protein breakdown induced by this hormonal environment are amplified by the relative inactivity of FT fibers, in fact creating a vicious circle. To support this contention, we demonstrated that the IgFI concentration which is lower in LSES girls living in Santa Cruz than in their counterparts of HSES is an explanatory factor for their lower P_{max} [10]. It has been hypothesized that this peptide could act on anaerobic power through the regulation of both muscle mass and muscle function.

All these effects of nutritional deprivation on skeletal muscle could well explain why anaerobic power, unlike aerobic power, is reduced in LSES children. However, it is questionable whether these results obtained under severe malnutrition can be extended to children suffering from marginal malnutrition. Because of ethical limitations, no data on muscle biopsies from these children are avalaible.

However, two observations give indirect information on muscle function in LSES children. Firstly, the same relationships in LSES and HSES children between [L] Wingate and the corresponding MP suggest an equal glycolytic activation during the test [21]. In contrast, it has been shown that severe nutritional deprivation reduces the concentrations of the key-regulating enzymes of the glycolysis (hexokinase, phosphofructokinase) and of the glycogenolysis (glycogen phosphatase and synthetase), and also lactate dehydrogenase activity. Secondly, FT subtype B fibers which are characterized by high contractile speed are probably preserved in LSES children because no difference in the optimal velocity (V_{opt}) for which P_{max} is obtained is found between HSES and LSES boys and girls [7, 8]. Conversely, a significantly lower optimal force (F_{opt}; which corresponds to V_{opt}) in malnourished children (–7% in boys [8] and –16% in girls [7]) could indicate a preferential alteration of FT subtype A fibers.

Besides a possible impaired muscle function, the lower anaerobic performance in LSES groups may result from a more limited coordination and technique in delivering external power during short-term exercise on a cycle ergometer. The HSES children have greater access to cycles and are probably more experienced cyclists than LSES children. Girls especially experience difficulties cycling in a coordinated way and this could explain why, when combined with a lesser degree of motivation and sense of competition, they have a performance markedly lower than boys.

Performances and Growth

The data which are only available in La Paz and Clermont-Ferrand in well-nourished boys between the ages of 7 and 15 indicate the following. (1) The altitude of La Paz does not modify the increase in $\dot{V}O_{2max}$ (liters/min) normally observed during this period [from 18]. The slopes of the relationships between these two parameters are the same at HA and LA. This increase is 0.184 liter/min/year while $\dot{V}O_{2max}$ at HA remains systematically lower than at LA (–0.45 liter/min). Expressed by body weight, no significant changes with age are found at LA as has been reported in numerous studies at sea level. The same result is observed in La Paz (fig. 3). (2) The rise in anaerobic performance with growth is not affected by chronic hypoxia (fig. 4, 5). P_{max} (in W/kg body weight) increases by 70–80% in boys between 7 and 15 years of age at both altitudes [18]. Similarly the same rates of enhancement at HA and LA are observed for MP (by a mean of 0.5 W/kg body weight a year). These increases are close to those reported by other authors in boys at sea level.

Summary and Conclusions

In this study, the effects of altitude and malnutrition on physical performances have been reviewed indicating the following. (1) Bolivian children living at the altitude of 3,600 m in La Paz have reduced aerobic performance irrespective of their socioeconomic and nutritional status. In contrast, at both altitudes marginal malnutrition does not alter $\dot{V}O_{2max}$ when adjusted to body dimension. (2) The altitude of 3,600 m does not modify anaerobic performances involving mainly alactic metabolism. When exercise duration is longer than a few seconds, anaerobic performances are reduced by chronic hypoxia because of a lower glycolytic and perhaps aerobic participation in energy contribution. This is true whatever the socioeconomic and nutritional status. (3) In contrast to aerobic performance, a marginal malnutrition reduces anaerobic performances at HA as well as at LA, expressed either in absolute terms or adjusted for body dimensions. An impaired muscle function as a direct or indirect consequence of malnutrition is suggested. (4) In Santa Cruz, tropical climate and other environmental factors such as parasitosis, cultural and psychological factors may have contributed to weaken performances in children from low and upper socioeconomic class, especially in girls as compared to their respective European counterparts. (5) Finally when the children are well-fed, the increase in $\dot{V}O_{2max}$ and anaerobic power during growth is the same in Bolivian boys living in La Paz as in lowland French boys.

References

1 Obert P, Fellmann N, Falgairette G, Bedu M, Van Praagh E, Kemper H, Post B, Spielvogel H, Tellez V, Quintela A, Coudert J: The importance of socioeconomic and nutritional conditions rather than altitude on the physical growth of prepubertal Andean highland boys. Ann Hum Biol 1994; 21/2:145–154.
2 de Onis M, Montero C, Akre J, Clugston G: The worldwide magnitude of protein-energy malnutrition: An overview from the WHO Global Database on child growth. Bull WHO 1993;71: 703–712.
3 Post GB, Kemper HCG, Welten DC, Coudert J: Dietary pattern and growth of 10–12-year-old Bolivian girls and boys: Relation between altitude and socioeconomic status. Am J Hum Biol 1997; 9:51–62.
4 Greksa LP, Haas JD: Physical growth and maximal work capacity in preadolescent boys at high altitude. Hum Biol 1982;54:677–695.
5 Greksa LP, Haas JD, Leatherman TL, Spielvogel H, Paz Zamora M, Paredes-Fernandez L, Moreno-Black G: Maximal aerobic power in trained youths at high altitude. Ann Hum Biol 1982;9:201–209.
6 Greksa LP, Spielvogel H, Paredes-Fernandez L: Maximal exercise capacity in adolescent European and Amerindian high-altitude natives. Am J Phys Anthropol 1985;67:209–216.
7 Blonc S, Fellmann N, Bedu M, Falgairette G, de Jonge R, Obert P, Beaune B, Spielvogel H, Tellez W, Quintela A, San Miguel JL, Coudert J: Effect of altitude and socio-economic status on VO_{2max} and anaerobic power in prepubertal Bolivian girls. J Appl Physiol 1996;80:2002–2008.
8 Obert P, Bedu M, Fellmann N, Falgairette G, Beaune B, Quintela A, Van Praagh E, Spielvogel H, Kemper H, Post B, Parent G, Coudert J: Effect of chronic hypoxia and socioeconomic status on VO_{2max} and anaerobic power of Bolivian boys. J Appl Physiol 1993;74:888–896.
9 Slooten J, Kemper HCG, Post GB, Lujan C, Coudert J: Habitual physical activity in 10 to 12-year-old Bolivian boys. The relation between altitude and socio-economic status. Int J Sports Med 1994; 15(suppl 2):S106-S111.
10 Beaune B, Blonc S, Fellmann N, Bedu M, Coudert J: Serum insulin-like growth factor I and physical performance in prepubertal Bolivian girls of a high and low socio-economic status. Eur J Appl Physiol 1997;76:98–102.
11 Fellmann N, Coudert J, Spielvogel H, Bedu M, Obert P, Falgairette G, Van Praagh E: Physical fitness of children resident at high altitude in Bolivia. Int J Sports Med 1992;13(suppl 1):S92-S95.

12 Falgairette G, Bedu M, Fellmann N, Spielvogel H, Van Praagh E, Obert P, Coudert J: Evaluation of physical fitness from field tests at high altitude in circumpubertal boys: Comparison with laboratory data. Eur J Appl Physiol 1994;69:36–43.
13 Andersen KL: The effect of altitude variation on the physical performance capacity of Ethiopian men. II. Development of physical performance during adolescence; in Seliger V (ed): Physical Fitness. Prague, Charles University, 1973, pp 34–36.
14 de Jonge R, Bedu M, Fellmann N, Blonc S, Spielvogel H, Coudert J: Effect of anthropometric characteristics and socio-economic status on physical performances of pre-pubertal children living in Bolivia at low altitude. Eur J Appl Physiol 1996;74:367–374.
15 Spurr GB, Reina JC: Maximum oxygen consumption in marginally malnourished Colombian boys and girls 6–16 years of age. Am J Hum Biol 1989;1:11–19.
16 Satyanarayana K, Naidu AN, Rao BSN: Nutritional deprivation in childhood and the body size, activity, and physical work capacity of young boys. Am J Clin Nutr 1979;32:1769–1775.
17 Bedu M, Coudert J: High altitude and anaerobic performance during growth; in Van Praagh E (ed): Pediatric Anaerobic Performance. Champaign, Human Kinetics 1998, pp 337–352.
18 Bedu M, Fellmann N, Spielvogel H, Falgairette G, Van Praagh E, Coudert J: Force-velocity and 30-second Wingate tests in boys at high and low altitudes. J Appl Physiol 1991;70:1031–1037.
19 Blonc S, Falgairette G, Bedu M, Fellmann N, Spielvogel H, Coudert J: The effect of acute hypoxia at low altitude and acute normoxia at high altitude on performance during a 30-s Wingate test in children. Int J Sports Med 1994;15:403–407.
20 Fellmann N, Bedu M, Spielvogel H, Falgairette G, Van Praagh E, Coudert J: Oxygen debt in submaximal and supramaximal exercise in children at high and low altitude. J Appl Physiol 1986;60/1:209–215.
21 Fellmann N, Beaune B, Coudert J: Blood lactate after maximal and supramaximal exercise in 10- to 12-year-old Bolivian boys: Effects of altitude and socio-economic status. Int J Sports Med 1994;15(suppl 2):S90-S95.
22 Fellmann N, Bedu M, Spielvogel H, Falgairette G, Van Praagh E, Jarrige JF, Coudert J: Anaerobic metabolism during pubertal development at high altitude. J Appl Physiol 1988;64:1382–1386.
23 Fellmann N, Coudert J: Malnutrition and anaerobic performance in children, in Van Praagh E (ed): Pediatric Anaerobic Performance. Champaign, Human Kinetics 1998, pp 319–335.

Nicole Fellmann, Laboratory of Physiology and Sports Biology, Faculty of Medicine,
Place H. Dunant, F–63001 Clermont-Ferrand (France)

Nutritional Status, Physical Fitness and Physical Activity in Children and Youth in Maputo (Mozambique)

António Prista

Faculdade de Ciencias de EF e Desporto, Maputo, Mozambique

Introduction

Studies of African children and youth have consistently shown lower rates of growth than international standards of reference [1–4]. This trend has also been observed in Mozambicans [5, 6]. Assuming that a deviation of so-called normal growth indicates a nutritional deficiency, anthropometric norms have been used as an indicator of nutritional status of a population, particularly children [7]. However, the classification of the nutritional status of a child, from the centile position that he/she occupies in relation to others, has been a controversial issue [8–10]. Despite the recognition that nutrition plays an important role in growth rates, the use of NCHS norms as the worldwide references to define a child as either normally nourished or malnourished has been shown to lead to incorrect conclusions [11]. The controversy about this topic has several bases which include the interaction of genetic and environmental factors affecting growth, the advantages and disadvantages of small stature, and the concept of nutritional status [12–14]. Some authors argue that it would be more useful to interpret anthropometric data related to nutritional status as the meaning it has for the health and well-being of a person who lives in a particular environment, which can be measured by the capacity to perform work and resist diseases [10]. In this way, one could consider physical activity (PA) and physical fitness as factors and/or indicators of nutritional status.

In order to test the relevance of nutritional anthropometric indicators of nutritional status for physical fitness and PA, we conducted a cross-sectional

Table 4. F and p values resulting from factorial ANOVA of comparison of AC among nutritional groups using age as covariant

Activity group	Boys		Girls	
	F	p	F	p
Households	0.73	0.53	0.57	0.63
Games	2.62	0.05	0.59	0.61
Sports	2.97	0.03	2.44	0.07
Walking time per day	1.89	0.13	0.96	0.41
Total activity	2.25	0.08	0.30	0.82

In all cases age has a significant effect, but no interaction was observed.

Table 5. F and p values resulting from factorial ANOVA of comparison of fitness tests among nutritional groups using age as covariant

Fitness test	Boys		Girls	
	F	p	F	p
Handgrip	21.8	0.000	13.0	0.000
Sit and reach	1.10	0.34	0.09	0.96
Sit-up	1.60	0.18	4.24	0.006
5 × 10-meter run	4.99	0.002	0.46	0.70
1,600-meter run	0.29	0.82	1.68	0.17
2,400-meter run	0.28	0.04	2.77	0.04

In all cases age has a significant effect.

30.5% of the girls exhibited some kind of malnutrition while 53.8 and 69.5% of boys and girls, respectively, were in the identified normal range of anthropometric values (table 3).

Comparisons of levels of PA in the nutritional groups were made according to the type of activity (table 4). With the exception of participation in sports for boys, the nutritional classification does not explain any variation in the level of activity. This means that this classification does not affect the PA habits of those children and youth.

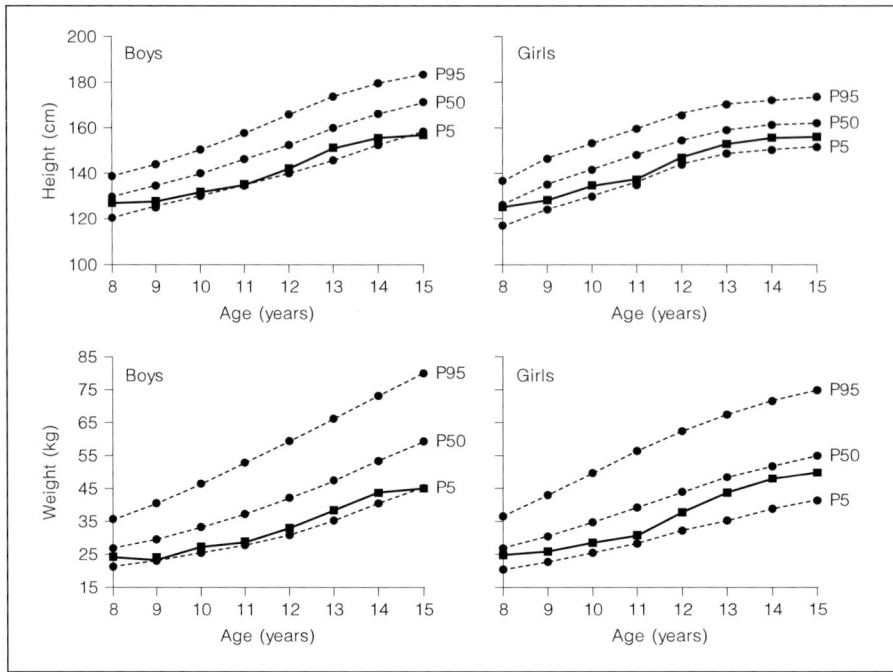

Fig. 1. Means of height and weight by sex as a function of age plotted under normative values adopted by the World Health Organization. —— = Maputo; - - - - = NCHS; P = percentile.

analysis was followed by a post-hoc Scheffé F test to verify differences by age group, particularly when differences were significant.

Since three different criteria are normally used to define cutoff points (the 3rd percentile, the minus-two standard deviation and 85th percentile of the median) the analysis was preceded by testing the proportional agreement of the three criteria. Using the kappa coefficient (that is, the proportion of agreement corrected for change of correct classification) a low agreement, in some cases, is observed (table 2). This means that, in some cases, we are violating the cross validity of these cutoff points. As this was more evident between the percentage of median and the two others, the use of one of the latter was decided upon. Arbitrarily we used the 3rd percentile as the criterion for the classification of the groups.

Results

Means of height and weight of Maputo students fall below the 50th percentile and close to the 5th percentile of the NCHS norms (fig. 1). Using the procedure described in the methodology section, 46.2% of the boys and

Table 2. Proportion of agreement and K coefficient between three different criteria according to classified nutritional status in Maputo children and youth

Indicator	Criterion on comparison	%	K
Weight for age	Z score × percentile	95	0.80
	Z score × % of median	37	0.08
	Percentile × % median	42	0.12
Weight for height	Z score × percentile	98	0.66
	Z score × % of median	79	0.13
	Percentile × % median	80	0.25
Height for age	Z score × percentile	96	0.85
	Z score × % of median	97	0.88
	Percentile × % median	93	0.75

Table 3. Number and percentage of subjects in each nutritional group

Nutritional group	Boys		Girls	
	n	%	n	%
Normal	134	53.8	198	69.5
Wasted	29	11.7	17	6.0
Stunted	28	11.7	34	11.9
Wasted and stunted	58	23.2	36	12.6

strength and 10 × 5-meter shuttle run were added. On the basis of three anthropometric indicators of nutritional status (weight for age, height for age, weight for height) the sample was classified into four groups, namely group 1 (normal): those who had height for age and weight for height above the cutoff points, group 2 (wasted): those who had height for age within the normal range and weight for height below the cutoff point, group 3 (stunted): those who had height for age below the cutoff point and weight for height in the normal range, and group 4 (wasted and stunted): those who had both indicators below the cutoff points. Because NCHS norms for weight for height do not give information above 137 cm of height, the indicator weight for age instead of weight for height was considered in those who had height over this value. To test the effect of the nutritional classification on PA and fitness, the results of PA and physical fitness were compared by sex through the factorial ANOVA procedure, with the fitness test score as the dependent variable and the nutritional group as the factor. To control the effect of age, this indicator was input as a covariant. This

Table 1. Descriptive statistics of Maputo children and youth: height and weight by age and sex (means ± SD)

Age years	Boys			Girls		
	n	height cm	weight kg	n	height cm	weight kg
8	27	127.0 ± 5.2	23.9 ± 3.2	34	125.1 ± 6.4	24.3 ± 4.1
9	22	127.7 ± 4.9	23.4 ± 3.0	35	128.3 ± 5.2	25.5 ± 3.6
10	39	132.2 ± 4.2	27.1 ± 3.7	37	134.8 ± 6.7	28.5 ± 4.5
11	39	135.5 ± 5.9	28.6 ± 4.0	44	137.3 ± 6.2	30.7 ± 4.7
12	35	142.5 ± 7.0	33.2 ± 5.3	28	147.3 ± 6.9	37.4 ± 6.1
13	41	151.7 ± 9.3	38.4 ± 6.2	42	152.8 ± 6.5	43.6 ± 7.0
14	19	156.1 ± 9.3	43.8 ± 7.1	37	156.1 ± 5.8	47.9 ± 6.6
15	28	157.2 ± 5.9	44.9 ± 6.2	28	156.1 ± 5.8	50.0 ± 7.4

study with Maputo children and youth. Although the majority of the studies on nutritional status are undertaken with children under 5, given the greater mortality and morbidity in this age range, it was assumed that the survivors of a malnutrition process during infancy could be affected by potential injuries which have long-term repercussions on their genetic potential. Because very few studies have been carried out with school children in this area, the present study used this specific population.

Methods

A cross-sectional sample of 593 students, 277 boys and 316 girls, 8–15 years of age was selected from three different regions of Maputo. Age was established according to both the self-reported age of the students, and the official documents of the school. Subjects were divided into four age groups: 8–9, 10–11, 12–13 and 14–15 years. The number of subjects and descriptive statistics of somatic characteristics of the sample are shown in table 1. Fifty-nine subjects (27 boys and 32 girls) were excluded from the analysis due to absence on several days of the tests.

Height, weight, PA and physical fitness were assessed between August and November 1992. All students had a medical examination and were considered clinically healthy. Habitual PA was assessed by a questionnaire which was conceptualized and validated for this specific population and described elsewhere [6, 15]. Each subject was assigned an activity coefficient (AC). For practical reasons, activities were grouped by type, namely indoor and outdoor household tasks, sports, outdoor games and walking. Physical fitness was assessed using the health-related fitness test battery (AAHPERD, 1980), which is composed of the sit and reach test, sit-ups, 1,600-meter run (8–11 years) and 2,400-meter run (12–15 years). Handgrip

A post-hoc examination revealed that the significant differences in sports participation in boys are due to the higher level of AC of the normal group. Comparisons between fitness test results in the nutritional groups show no differences in sit and reach and 1,600-meter run tests in both sex groups. The significant differences are in the handgrip and 2,400-meter run in both sexes, in the 10 × 5-meter run for boys and in the sit-ups for girls (table 5).

A post-hoc examination showed that the normal group performed significantly better in the handgrip in all age groups, but worse in the 2,400-meter run. Differences in sit-ups for girls, and 10 × 5-meter run for boys are due to the significantly better performances of the so-called well-off groups. These differences are not consistent in all age groups.

Discussion

Although the rate of growth and the nutritional status have been extensively studied in children's early years, the study of African school age population is still insufficient. In general, when compared to international standards of reference, the average body dimensions of African children and youth are consistently inferior [1–5], which was also observed in the present study with Mozambican children and youth. It was suggested that the pattern of growth after 5 years of age is homogeneous for the whole of sub-Saharan Africa [1]. However, Van Loon [11] observed that inside Africa, ethnic group differences of populations were more important than group variance according to sex, which suggests that if one calls for sex-specific standards then it would be more important to use ethnic-specific norms. Unfortunately, this study was carried out with children under 5 and the results cannot be generalized for school-aged children.

The use of anthropometry as an indicator of nutritional status has become a controversial issue, particularly when an international norm of reference is being adopted to classify nutritional status. Although the influence of the nutrition process on growth is a well-known fact, caution has been suggested regarding the simple classification of malnourished individuals from the percentile criterion of NCHS norms given that the factors that contribute to the height of an individual are not limited to the nutrition [11, 16–19]. The present study tested the meaning of the anthropometric nutritional classification for habitual PA and physical fitness, assuming that a deficiency in nutrition should affect the capacity to perform work and daily tasks.

With the exception for sports participation and games in boys, no differences were found in PA habits between the so-called normal group and well-off groups. Prista et al. [15], in a study with the same population, compared

Table 6. Comparison of relative strength between the nutritional groups by sex and age group

	Age group years	Nutritional group				
		normal	wasted	stunted	wasted/stunted	p
Boys	8–9	0.51 ± 0.08	0.48 ± 0.07		0.44 ± 0.09	0.15
	10–11	0.58 ± 0.11	0.45 ± 0.15	0.51 ± 0.09	0.54 ± 0.07	0.03
	12–13	0.57 ± 0.10	0.61 ± 0.09	0.58 ± 0.07	0.59 ± 0.10	0.77
	14–15	0.67 ± 0.11	0.70 ± 0.04	0.66 ± 0.15	0.66 ± 0.10	0.89
Girls	8–9	0.47 ± 0.10	0.48 ± 0.05	0.40 ± 0.15	0.46 ± 0.10	0.46
	10–11	0.69 ± 0.26	0.51 ± 0.21	0.64 ± 0.28	0.66 ± 0.18	0.31
	12–13	0.56 ± 0.08	0.63 ± 0.04	0.55 ± 0.06	0.59 ± 0.08	0.33
	14–15	0.59 ± 0.07	0.58 ± 0.07	0.58 ± 0.12	0.60 ± 0.04	0.88

Values represent means ± SD (kg F/kg). p values of one-way ANOVA as shown.

the body size and PA habits among socioeconomic groups. They found that although the underprivileged children had significant deficits in their attained height, they exhibited a higher level of activity due to the higher demands of survival activities (such as walking and carrying) and participation in recreational active games. Whilst an early childhood reduction of activity in order to maintain homeostasis was reported among the malnourished [20–22], several studies with school-age populations do not observe such a reduction [23, 24]. Peer pressure, survival needs and growth retardation are cited as the main reason for this finding [12, 25]. Taking into account studies done with school-age Mozambican populations [15, 26], one could also suggest a strong cultural determinant, because poor children of Mozambique use to play and dance outside rather then watch TV or play video games. Only a very small number of the sample (9%) participated in formal sports and they were representative of the privileged group who were also taller. Results suggest that if the cutoff points suggested to classify malnutrition are assumed, one would conclude that a nutritional deficit does not affect PA levels in this population.

It is reasonable to suggest that the normal nutritional group would perform better in physical fitness tasks. However, the only significant and consistent performance in the different nutritional age and sex groups studied was in the handgrip strength test. This result was expected as handgrip tests are muscle mass-dependent and this was the criterion used to form the groups. When the analyses are made using relative strength (that is, dividing the score by body weight), the significance disappears (table 6).

Other differences found (2,400-meter run, sit-ups in boys and 5 × 10-meter run in girls) were due to the better performances of the so-called well-off groups. Prista et al. [15] observed that when body size was not a determinant for a given test, Mozambican children and youth performed better than their peers from several developed countries. Characterizing the habitual PA of this population they suggested that these differences could be caused by a more active lifestyle. Despite a lower body height, the underprivileged children performed significantly better than the privileged ones from the same ethnic origin. Thus, one could hypothesize that the difference in the 10 × 5-meter and endurance run could be a function of lifestyle and not of the nutritional status.

The few studies completed on Africa school-age children concerning physical fitness generally show that absolute levels of maximal oxygen consumption, muscle strength and anaerobic power fall below the norms of developed countries [Bénéfice, unpubl. data]. However, if one takes into account the difference in body mass, motor performance tends to be equal or even higher [4, 15, 27–29]. Interpretation and controversy about advantages and disadvantages of being average or small have been polemic. Stini [12] has suggested that a lower growth rate is an adaptive response to the adverse conditions leading to less need for feeding. Additionally some authors have suggested that people from developing countries are mechanically more efficient than their taller peers from developed countries. This notion was rejected by studies where muscle efficiency was compared between normal and 'marginally' malnourished children and youth [14, 30]. The advantages of being small were also contested by the argument that in countries where manual labor plays an important role in productivity, the absolute capacity to perform work would be more important than the relative one [24].

The discussion of this topic has led to the claim that the acceptance of the adaptation theory could constitute a way of perpetuating and justifying social imbalances, assuming that the stunted condition reflects a social inequality [13]. However, results from some studies suggested that the use of the NCHS norms as the guideline to classify malnutrition (and consequently intervention) would lead to needs of emergency intervention in a higher percentage of African children, most of them were found to be clinically healthy [11].

This study has several limitations since only fitness and PA habits were taken into account. No data about other important parameters, such as those related to resistance to diseases, were observed. Moreover, studies on the school-age African population are scarce which prevents more consistent conclusions. Taking into account these limitations, the results are in agreement with those who suggest caution in using NCHS norms as a criterion to classify the nutritional state. Van Loon [11] has underlined that 'to identify a malnourished child for treatment among his local peers is a procedure which is totally different from the comparison between several population groups' [11]. The claim for local comparisons has been justified in the present study although the operative and cost implications still remain an impairment.

Summary and Conclusions

Two hundred seventy-seven boys and 316 girls, 8–15 years of age selected from three different regions of Maputo, were examined cross-sectionally. The subjects were subdivided according to age, gender and nutritional status (group 1 = normal, 2 = wasted, 3 = stunted, 4 = wasted and stunted). With the exception of participation in sports for boys, nutritional classification did not explain any variation in the PA level. Comparisons between results of fitness testing showed no differences in sit and reach and 1,600-meter run tests as regards the nutritional status of children and youth. Significantly better results were shown in handgrip strength measurements in group 1 in both genders, and in the 10×5-meter run in boys and in sit-ups in girls. On the other hand, the results in the 2,400-meter run were worse in group 1. The differences were not completely consistent in all age groups.

These data seem to indicate that in spite of the smaller body size of the underprivileged children their performance in some disciplines was better. The differences in handgrip strength can be explained by higher body weight and larger muscle mass of subjects in group 1; the differences in 10×5-meter run and endurance could be a function of lifestyle in children with different nutritional and social statuses. These findings were in agreement with previous studies which showed that when body size was not a determinant for a given test, Mozambican children and youth performed better than their peers from several developed countries. The use of body size as a decisive indicator of nutritional status and positive health is thus controversial, especially when using the international reference values for children of different ethnic backgrounds and from various parts of the world. Functional testing could help to differentiate and define more precisely the nutritional and health status during growth as related to the environment.

References

1 Eveleth PB, Tanner JM: Worldwide Variation in Human Growth; in International Biological Program 8. Cambridge, Cambridge University Press, 1976.
2 Corlett JT: Growth of urban schoolchildren in Botswana. Ann Hum Biol 1986;13:73–82.
3 Cameron N, Hiernaux J, Jarman S, Marshall WA, Tanner JM, Withehouse RH: Anthropometry; in Weisner JS, Lourie JA (eds): Practical Human Biology. New York, Academic Press, 1981.
4 Nkiama E: Croissance, maturation osseuse et perfomance physiques des enfants scolarisés zaïrois de Bunia âgés de 6 à 20 ans. Leuven, Katholieke Universiteit Leuven, 1993.
5 Martins DC: Dinâmica do crescimento e desenvolvimento da criança em Moçambique; Dissertacao de Doutoramento, Faculdade de Medicina da Universidade de Coimbra, 1968.
6 Prista A: Influence of Physical Activity and Socioeconomic Factors on the Components of Health Related Fitness in Mozambican Schoolchildren; doctoral dissertation thesis University of Porto, 1994.
7 WHO Working Group: Use and interpretation of anthropometric indicators of nutritional status. Bull World Organ 1986;64:929–941.
8 Habicht JP, Matorell R, Yarbrough C, Malina RM, Klein RE: Height and weight standards for preschool children: How relevant are ethnic differences in growth potential? Lancet 1974;i:611–614.
9 Goldstein H, Tanner JM: Ecological considerations on the use of anthropometry to assess nutritional status. Lancet 1980;i:582–585.
10 Cameron N: Measurement issues related to the anthropometric assessement of nutritional status; in Himes J (ed): Anthropometric Assessment of Nutritional Status. New York, Wiley-Liss, 1991, pp 347–364.
11 Van Loon A: Epidemiology of Malnutrition in Developing Countries: A Novel Anthropometrical Screening Strategy. Leuven, Katholieke Universiteit Leuven, 1987.
12 Stini WA: Adaptive strategies of human populations under nutritional stress; in Watts ES, Johnston FE, Lasker GW (eds): Biosocial Interrelations in Population Adaptation. The Hague, Mouton, 1975, pp 19–41.
13 Martorell R, Mendonza F, Castillo R: Poverty and stature in children; in Waterlow JC (ed): Linear Growth Retardation in Less Developed Countries. New York, Raven Press, 1988, vol 14, pp 57–73.
14 Spurr GB: Body size, physical work capacity and productivity in hard work: Is bigger better?; in Waterlow JC (ed): Linear Growth Retardation in Less Developed Countries. New York, Raven Press, 1988, vol 14, pp 215–224.
15 Prista A, Marques AT, Maia AJR: Relationship between physical activity, socioeconomic status, and physical fitness of 8–15 year old youth from Mozambique. Am J Hum Biol 1997;9:449–457.
16 Malina RM: Socio-cultural influences of physical activity and performance. Bull Soc Belge Anthropol Préhist 1983;94:155–176.
17 Eveleth PB: Population differences in growth: Environmental and genetic factors; in Falkner F, Tanner JM (eds): Human Growth 3. New York, Plenum Press, 1986, pp 221–239.
18 Waterlow JC: Observations on the natural history of stunting; in Waterlow JC (ed): Linear Growth Retardation in Less Developed Countries. New York, Raven Press, 1988, vol 14, pp 1–17.
19 Cameron N: Human growth, nutrition and health in sub-Saharan Africa. Yearb Phys Anthropol 1991;34:211–250.
20 Chavez A, Martinez C, Bourges H: Nutrition and development of infants from poor rural areas. II. Nutritional level and physical activity. Nutr Rep Int 1972;5:139.
21 Rutishauer IHE, Whitehead RG: Energy intake and expenditure in 1–3-year-old Ugandan children living in a rural environment. Br J Nutr 1972;28:145–152.
22 Torun B, Viteri FE: Energy requirements of pre-schoolchildren and effects of varying energy intakes on protein metabolism; in Torun B, Young VR, Rand WM (eds): Protein-Energy Requirements of Developing Countries: Evaluation of New Data, 1981, suppl 5.
23 Satayanarayana MB, Naidu AN, Rao BSN: Nutritional deprivation in childhood and the body size, activity and physical work capacity of young boys. Am J Clin. Nutr 1979;32:1769–1775.
24 Spurr GB, Reina JC, Barac-Nieto M: Marginal malnutrition in school-aged Colombian boys: Metabolic rate and estimated daily energy expenditure. Am J Clin Nutr 1986;44:113–126.

25 Spurr GB, Reina JC: Influence of dietary intervention on artificially increased activity in marginally undernourished Colombian boys. Eur J Clin Nutr 1988;42:835–846.
26 Prista A, Guedes G: O Jogo em Moçambique: Uma introdução ao seu estudo; in Bento J, Marques A (eds): Actas do II Congresso de Educação Física dos Países de Língua Portuguesa, 1991, vol 2, pp 419–431.
27 Areskog NH, Selinus R, Vahlsqvist B: Physical work capacity and nutritional status in Ethiopian male children and young adults. Am J Clin Nutr 1969;22:471–479.
28 Ghesquière, Eeckels R: Health, physical development and fitness of primary schoolchildren in Kinshasa; in Ilmarinen J, Välimaki I (eds): Children and Sport: Pediatric Work Physiology. Berlin, Springer, 1981, pp 18–30.
29 Malina RM: Motor development and performance of children and youth in undernourished populations; in Katch FI (ed): Sport, Health and Nutrition. Champaign, Human Kinetics Books, 1986, pp 213–225.
30 Spurr GB, Barac-Nieto M, Reina JC, Ramirez R: Marginal malnutrition in school-aged Colombian boys: Efficiency of treadmill walking in submaximal exercise. Am J Clin Nutr 1984;39:452–459.

Dr. António Prista, Faculdade de Ciencias de EF e Desporto,
CP 2107, Maputo (Mozambique)

Evaluation of Physical Status of Children Living in the Zones of Influence of Small Doses of Radiation after the Chernobyl Accident

K. Kozlova

Vinnitsa State Pedagogic Institute, Vinnitsa, Ukraine

Introduction

The most important goals in the promotion of physical health of a human being are relatively high absolute indices of bodily function and a high level of adaptability of the major systems [1–3]. A modern understanding of physical health is based on the complex of biosocial properties of an individual, and an active and effective functioning in the environment. One might contend that the wider the range of adaptive abilities of a human being, the quicker and better he or she may act under the conditions of a changing environment, the more effective he or she may be in both problem-solving and susceptibility to many illnesses. One of the most compelling and challenging questions of scientific and public interest is the question of the influence of radiation on human beings and the environment [4, 6]. There is currently considerable concern amongst the public worldwide about influence of radiation on human beings and especially on children [5, 7].

As a result of the accident at the Chernobyl electric power station, a unique and historical experience occurred, affecting numerous strata of the population, including children. More than 3 million citizens live in the territories polluted with radiation. A great number of radionuclides have been released into the atmosphere. During the accident, together with other radioactive fallouts, the amount of cesium-137 reached 1.9×10^6 C. The territory of the Ukraine had 6% of the cesium-137 fallout.

Accumulation of radionuclides in the human body may result in the development of disorders of different organs and systems. Children are believed to have been most affected by radionuclides, but the biological influence of small doses of radiation on the physical status of the growing child has not been studied comprehensively. The problem has only been addressed by different groups of researchers since 1990.

The normal growth and development of children and their predisposition to a health status are influenced by both genetic and environmental factors. But the action of radionuclides varies according to the level of physical maturity of the individual. For example, the half-life of cesium-137 for adults is 70–140 days (on average 110 days), whilst for children depending upon age and the level of metabolic processes, it takes from 20 to 50 days. The younger the organism, all other factors considered, the quicker are incorporated radionuclides eliminated from the body [1].

Subjects and Methods

In order to study the possible influence of small doses of radiation on the physical status of children, the current group project investigated more than 15,000 schoolchildren from 7 to 17 years of age who lived in the territories with a level of radioactive pollution of 1.5–8.0 C/km^2. Comparative data was collected on physical development and functional status of children using information collected in 1985 (before the Chernobyl accident). The study provides the opportunity to evaluate the differences in the physical condition of children living in the zone with increased levels of radiation. Research was performed at the first stage and allowed the authors to study the influence of small doses of radiation on the organisms of children in the first years after the accident.

Results

The physical development of children between 1985 and 1990 is represented in tables 1 and 2. There were no differences in body weight of boys aged 9, 10, 12, 13 and 14 years and of girls aged 8, 9, 10 and 16 years between 1985 and 1990. In contrast, the body height of boys aged 7, 8, 11, 15, 16 and 17 years and of girls aged 7, 12, 13, 14 and 15 years living in the zone of increased radiation was significantly greater ($p < 0.05$). Group means for body height are lower in 1990 for girls aged 9–11 and 17 years and for boys of 10 and 13–17 years. The data represent a progressive but irregular trend in the growth of youngsters aged 7–17 years. There is some evidence on the basis of these results for the stimulating action of small doses of radiation. The effect is short-lived, approximately 2–3 years, and this is followed by a sharp decline

Table 1. Height of children living in the zone of radioactive pollution (cm)

Age years	Boys		Girls	
	1990	1985	1990	1985
7	123.0 ($\pm$1.4)[a]	118.7 ($\pm$0.5)	125.1 ($\pm$1.1)[a]	117.3 ($\pm$0.6)
8	127.1 ($\pm$1.0)[a]	123.6 ($\pm$0.5)	127.8 ($\pm$1.0)	128.5 ($\pm$0.5)
9	133.1 ($\pm$1.1)	133.4 ($\pm$0.5)	132.3 ($\pm$1.1)	133.0 ($\pm$0.5)
10	132.7 ($\pm$3.5)	139.1 ($\pm$0.5)	135.5 ($\pm$1.8)	139.2 ($\pm$0.5)
11	144.1 ($\pm$1.0)[a]	139.8 ($\pm$0.5)	141.3 ($\pm$1.0)[a]	144.4 ($\pm$0.5)
12	149.1 ($\pm$1.4)	149.6 ($\pm$0.5)	150.9 ($\pm$1.3)[a]	146.5 ($\pm$0.6)
13	152.8 ($\pm$1.4)	153.6 ($\pm$0.6)	157.4 ($\pm$1.4)[a]	154.8 ($\pm$0.5)
14	159.5 ($\pm$1.4)	160.3 ($\pm$0.6)	161.4 ($\pm$0.9)[a]	156.5 ($\pm$0.6)
15	163.5 ($\pm$1.2)[a]	165.5 ($\pm$0.5)	163.1 ($\pm$1.0)[a]	161.1 ($\pm$0.5)
16	170.2 ($\pm$2.1)[a]	172.8 ($\pm$0.6)	163.2 ($\pm$1.1)	164.2 ($\pm$0.6)
17	173.0 ($\pm$2.6)[a]	175.0 ($\pm$0.6)	162.5 ($\pm$0.8)[a]	165.2 ($\pm$0.6)

[a] $p < 0.05$ vs. before.

Table 2. Body weight of children living in the zone of radioactive pollution (kg)

Age years	Boys		Girls	
	1990	1985	1990	1985
7	25.0 ($\pm$1.2)[a]	22.5 ($\pm$0.4)	25.8 ($\pm$1.0)[a]	22.3 ($\pm$0.4)
8	26.2 ($\pm$0.7)	28.1 ($\pm$0.4)	26.7 ($\pm$0.7)	27.8 ($\pm$0.4)
9	28.9 ($\pm$0.8)	30.2 ($\pm$0.4)	29.6 ($\pm$0.8)	29.9 ($\pm$0.4)
10	31.2 ($\pm$1.0)	34.6 ($\pm$0.6)	30.9 ($\pm$1.6)	33.5 ($\pm$0.6)
11	35.6 ($\pm$0.9)	35.3 ($\pm$0.5)	33.4 ($\pm$0.8)	39.2 ($\pm$0.7)
12	39.5 ($\pm$1.4)	41.2 ($\pm$0.7)	41.4 ($\pm$1.2)[a]	39.7 ($\pm$0.5)
13	44.2 ($\pm$1.2)[a]	41.6 ($\pm$0.4)	45.2 ($\pm$1.1)[a]	39.8 ($\pm$0.3)
14	46.7 ($\pm$1.7)	47.6 ($\pm$0.8)	51.2 ($\pm$1.6)[a]	49.2 ($\pm$0.9)
15	56.9 ($\pm$2.1)[a]	55.3 ($\pm$0.8)	51.8 ($\pm$1.6)	52.6 ($\pm$0.7)
16	60.3 ($\pm$0.7)	63.1 ($\pm$0.8)	54.1 ($\pm$0.7)	56.9 ($\pm$0.8)
17	61.8 ($\pm$3.5)	66.5 ($\pm$0.9)	55.3 ($\pm$2.7)	57.7 ($\pm$0.6)

[a] $p < 0.05$ vs. before.

in growth rates. This was confirmed by the observation of the groups of children during 3 years, 1990–1993.

In absolute terms, the growth rate of boys aged 7–10 years decreased from 5.7 to 3.5 cm and in girls of the same age from 4.4 to 3.2 cm. In percentage terms, the annual growth rate for body height for the same groups decreased

Table 3. Indices of functional development of children of 7–10 years of age living in the zone of radioactive pollution

Age years	Sex	Indices		
		spirometry (vital capacity) cm^3	pulse (bpm)	PWC$_{170}$ index
7	boys	1,379 ($\pm$66.7)	92.0 ($\pm$4.3)	43.1 ($\pm$1.0)
	girls	1,243 ($\pm$45.8)	91.1 ($\pm$4.1)	45.1 ($\pm$0.3)
8	boys	1,544 ($\pm$24.2)	90.0 ($\pm$1.3)	42.0 ($\pm$0.6)
	girls	1,432 ($\pm$55.6)	90.0 ($\pm$2.0)	42.1 ($\pm$0.8)
9	boys	1,859 ($\pm$29.0)	95.1 ($\pm$0.9)	43.2 ($\pm$0.7)
	girls	1,785 ($\pm$52.6)	95.4 ($\pm$1.9)	47.2 ($\pm$2.1)
10	boys	1,876 ($\pm$33.1)	94.9 ($\pm$1.2)	42.5 ($\pm$0.6)
	girls	1,790 ($\pm$25.0)	91.3 ($\pm$1.6)	41.4 ($\pm$1.8)

from 4.8 to 2.6 and 3.7 to 2.4%, respectively. In the 11- to 14-year age group, the annual growth rate in height of boys dropped from 3.7 to 2.4% and for girls from 6.7 to 2.5%.

Age changes in the body weight of children aged 7–17 years are characterized by the following. Boys aged 7, 13 and 15 years and girls of 7 and 12–14 years living in zones of action of small doses of radiation showed significant increases between the two measurement dates ($p<0.05$). For the rest of the age groups, 1985 values are higher than those for 1990. The mean annual weight gain for each group of boys in absolute indices is from 7 to 8 years 1.2 kg, from 8 to 9 years 2.7 kg, from 9 to 10 years 2.3 kg, from 10 to 11 years 4.4 kg, from 11 to 12 years 3.9 kg, from 12 to 13 years 4.7 kg, from 13 to 14 years 2.5 kg, from 14 to 15 years 10.2 kg, from 15 to 16 years 3.4 kg, from 16 to 17 years 1.5 kg. The girls have the following rates of gain in absolute indices: from 7 to 8 years 0.9 kg, from 8 to 9 years 2.9 kg, from 9 to 10 years 1.3 kg, from 10 to 11 years 2.5 kg, from 11 to 12 years 8.0 kg, from 12 to 13 years 3.8 kg, from 13 to 14 years 6.0 kg, from 14 to 15 years 0.6 kg, from 15 to 16 years 2.3 kg, and from 16 to 17 years 1.2 kg. These data quantify the delay in anticipated weight gains during these ages. In summary, junior schoolchildren were classified as follows. Body height characteristics were average in 70% of girls and 48% of boys whilst for body weight 44% of girls and 30% of boys showed an average development. The indices of functional status are presented in table 3.

Clinical observations and checkups revealed a range of deviations in the health condition of the children. In particular, enlargement of the thyroid gland of the first and second degree was found in 82% of the girls and 65% of the boys and lymphadenopathy was found in 63% of the girls and 21% of the boys. Dental caries was found in 79% of the girls and 72% of the boys whilst cardiopathy was evident in 26% of the girls and 21% of the boys.

The indices of spirometry (vital capacity) improved with age. Thus, boys of 7 years had a spirometry index of 1,379.0 cm^3 (± 66.7) whilst the girls' index was 1,243.0 cm^3 (± 48.8). During the period from 7 to 10 years, the index increased in absolute units for the boys by 497 cm^3 (36%) and for the girls by 547 cm^3 (44%). The mean annual rate of increase fluctuated from 11.9 to 20.4% for the boys and correspondingly from 15.2 to 24.6% for the girls. There were no sex differences in pulse rates for any age group.

Qualitatively, a positive trend may be observed with regard to the above indices. The number of children with indices 'lower than average' and 'low' decreased from 44 to 11.7% whilst the number of children with average levels increased from 52 to 62%. Research of a number of authors shows that an essential increase of vital capacity of lungs is noticed from 8 to 11 years. The boys are at an advantage over the girls. Under the influence of systematic training comprising physical exercise, the functional ability of the respiratory organs is increased.

The PWC_{170} index characterizes the level of physical work capacity for individuals. PWC_{170} declined with age from 7 to 9 years before increasing and then declining again at 10 years of age. PWC levels of all children were lower than expected. Observation of the children over a long period of time showed an increased vegetative liability, general weakness, drowsiness and apathy. The intensity of adaptation reactions of an organism in response to the action of small doses of radiation is initially increased, but reaches a maximum level. When exposed to a greater intensity of radiation for longer periods of time, the adaptation abilities of organisms become exhausted and subsequently replaced by compensation reactions.

A large amount of objective material regarding the physical abilities of children in this area has been collected. Analysis of these data makes it possible to suggest a definition of the main directions of the pedagogical influence on children in terms of physical training. It also points out the most susceptible periods for children with respect to learning different motor actions. The unique conditions of the environment as a result of increased radiation after the Chernobyl accident demand new approaches in the assessment of growth status and the physical training in order to facilitate an improvement of functions, without damaging the health of children.

An additional element of the current research was to evaluate the level of motor development of 8- to 10-year-olds who lived in zones with increased

Table 4. 20-meter running results (s)

Age years	Clean area		Polluted area	
	boys	girls	boys	girls
8	4.5 (± 0.8)	4.7 (± 0.12)	4.3 (± 0.05)	4.7 (± 0.06)
9	4.0 (± 0.08) [a]	4.5 (± 0.07)	4.8 (± 0.07)	4.5 (± 0.03)
10	4.4 (± 0.02)	5.3 (± 0.12)	4.8 (± 0.1)	4.6 (± 0.05) [a]

[a] $p < 0.05$ after vs. before.

radiation compared with an ecologically clean environment. Tests included a 20-meter run, throwing a tennis ball, throwing a weighted ball and a 6-min run. Each task was evaluated on a 5-point scale, 1 point for a low score and 5 points for a high score. For each separate task a 5-stage scale of evaluation was established: low (1 point), below average (2 points), average (3 points), above average (4 points) and high (5 points). The results obtained indicate that depending on the differences in their environment the development of major physical qualities in children is varied.

It was established that the level of the development of running abilities of schoolchildren living in different ecological zones is different (table 4). The data presented in table 4 gives a new understanding to the development of running speed abilities of 8- to 10-year-old children. One can see from these data that of 9- to 10-year-old children living in ecologically clean zones have higher indices than those of children living in the zone of increased radiation. Only the 8-year-old boys living in the polluted zone have an index of 4.3 ± 0.05 s versus 4.5 ± 0.08 s in the clean zone. Substantial differences have been established for the 9-year-old boys from the clean zone: 4.0 ± 0.08 s versus 4.8 ± 0.07 s ($t = 7.1$; $p < 0.001$). The 20-meter running index for 10-year-old girls in the clean zone was 5.3 ± 0.012 s and in the polluted area 4.6 ± 0.05 s ($t = 5.8$; $p < 0.05$). The 20-meter running index of the girls differs less with respect to age.

Data characterizing the development of force abilities are given in table 5. The 8- to 9-year-old boys from the clean zone have higher results as regards pushing the weighted ball than the boys of the same age living in the zone affected by small doses of radiation. No difference in pushing the weighted ball was found for the boys of 10 years. Reliable differences were found in the results of the 8-year-old boys ($t = 2.4$; $p < 0.05$). Results of 8-year-old girls in the clean zone were 1.9 ± 0.04 m and in the polluted zone 1.7 ± 0.04 m ($t = 3.2$; $p < 0.03$); results of the 9-year-old girls in the clean zone were 1.8 ± 0.2 m and

Table 5. Results of ball pushing (m)

Age years	Clean area		Polluted area	
	boys	girls	boys	girls
8	2.1 (±0.1) [a]	1.9 (±0.04) [a]	1.9 (±0.02) [a]	1.7 (±0.04)
9	3.5 (±0.01)	1.8 (±0.2)	3.2 (±0.1)	2.7 (±0.1) [a]
10	3.5 (±0.2)	2.5 (±0.1)	3.5 (±0.1)	3.0 (±0.2) [a]

[a] $p < 0.05$ after vs. before.

in the polluted zone 2.7 ± 0.1 m ($t = 3.7$; $p < 0.01$); results of the 10-year-old girls in the clean zone were 2.5 ± 0.1 m and in the polluted zone 3.0 ± 0.2 m ($t = 2.5$; $p < 0.05$). The increase of results in pushing the weighted ball by the 8- to 10-year-old boys from the clean zone was 66% and 84% from the polluted zone whereas results for the 8- to 10-year-old girls were 31% from the clean zone and 76% from the polluted zone.

Indices of the development of general endurance are presented in figure 1. Boys of 8–10 years of age living in the ecologically clean zone surpassed the boys living in the polluted zone in a 6-min running index. The result of 8-year-old boys from the clean zone was 866 ± 4.8 m compared to 700 ± 0.5 m for those from the polluted zone. At the age of 10, boys from the clean zone ran 978 m during 6 min in comparison to 898 m by the boys from the polluted zone. The boys from the clean zone have significantly higher results than the boys from the polluted zone ($t = 5.9$; $p < 0.05$). With respect to the development of general endurance, the girls from the polluted zone have the following indices: 8 years: 685 ± 0.06 m, 9 years: 696 ± 16.2, and 10 years: 824 ± 7.6 m. Better results were achieved by girls of 9 years from the clean zone: 916 ± 11.3 m. The girls living in the clean zone had significantly higher results than girls living in the zone of increased radiation. The endurance capacity is the basis of the function of the aerobic system. It is known that people with a low level of aerobic function often have a greater tendency to be affected by illnesses such as hypertension and obesity. A greater developed level of endurance provides the capacity to sustain work for longer periods of time.

The ability to hit a goal directly is expressed by the results of tennis ball throwing (table 6). The best results in hitting the goal were achieved by the 10-year-old boys from the polluted zone: 18.5 ± 0.9 points. Eight-year-old boys from the same zone showed lower results. The best results achieved by 9-year-old boys were decreased by nearly 30% compared to the age of 10. A similar

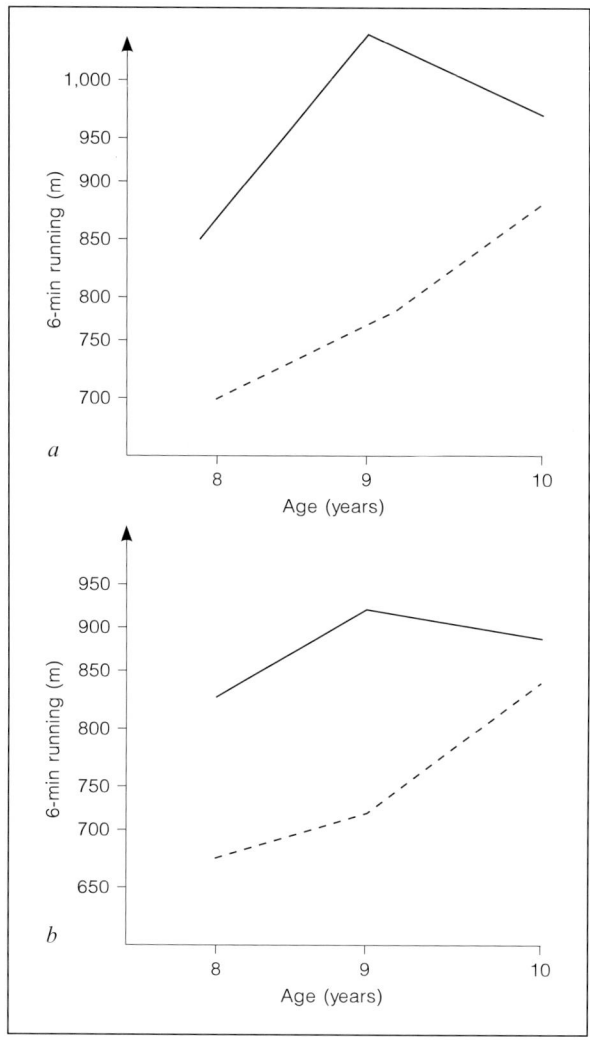

Fig. 1. Age changes of 6-min running performance of 8- to 10-year-old boys (*a*) and girls (*b*) from clean (—) and polluted (- - -) zones.

tendency was found in this index for the girls from the clean zone. The girls living in the zone of increased radiation displayed significantly better results at the ages of 8 and 10. A higher developmental level of coordination ability allows an individual to quickly practice and master new movements, and to rationally and systematically apply the available store of movement practice with respect to individual levels of physical development. Existing coordination

Table 6. Results of tennis ball throwing (points)

Age years	Clean area		Polluted area	
	boys	girls	boys	girls
8	11.6 ($\pm$0.8)	7.3 ($\pm$1.2)	16.8 ($\pm$0.4)[a]	14.7 ($\pm$0.5)[a]
9	16.5 ($\pm$1.0)[a]	20.0 ($\pm$1.2)	13.3 ($\pm$0.8)	17.6 ($\pm$1.2)
10	12.7 ($\pm$0.6)	9.1 ($\pm$0.4)	18.5 ($\pm$0.9)[a]	12.3 ($\pm$1.4)

[a] $p<0.05$ after vs. before.

ability provides a solid ground for the development and formation of many new skills and actions.

With respect to the developmental level of deftness (throwing of a rubber ball), differences are observed in the children from different ecological zones. Only 8-year-old children have identical results. It has been established that these results improve with age. Accordingly, 10-year-old boys from the polluted zone had a higher result, 24.8 ± 2.3 versus 19.0 ± 1.0 m of the boys from the clean zone. Reliable differences have been established with this index for the age of 9 and 10. In school-age boys and girls, there are two periods of increase and decrease in the improvement rates of results: from 7 to 9 and 14 to 16 years for the boys, and from 7 to 8 and 12 to 13 years for the girls. A comparison of the age and sex differences of children from different ecological zones showed, in most cases, a substantial superiority of the children living in an ecologically clean zone.

Discussion

Qualitative evaluation of the results allowed the establishment not only of absolute indices in tests, but also the establishment of developmental levels of physical ability. The level of development of speed ability is expressed in the following data: 50% of 8-year-old boys from the clean zone had a level above the average, 10% average, 20% high and 20% below average. Boys of the same age from the ecologically polluted zone had the following levels: 48% above average, 22% high, 26% average and 4% below average. Among the 9-year-old boys from the clean zone, 41% had a level above average, 31% high, 12.5 average and 12.5 below average. Boys of the same age from the polluted zone had the following levels: 47% below average, 35% low and 18% average. Among the 10-year-old boys from the clean zone, 60% had a low

Table 7. Level of development of endurance (6-min running test)

Zone	8-year-old											9-year-old											10-year-old											
	boys						girls						boys						girls						boys						girls				
	h	h/a	a	l/a	l		h	h/a	a	l/a	l		h	h/a	a	l/a	l		h	h/a	a	l/a	l		h	h/a	a	l/a	l		h	h/a	a	l/a	l
Clean			100						100				87		13					19	75	6					100					10	50		40
Polluted				96	4					30	70				47	53						30	70				43	50	70				29	71	

h = High; h/a = high average; a = average; l/a = low average; l = low.

level of speed development ability and 40% a high level whilst 71% of boys from the polluted zone had a level below average and 20% a low level.

The level of speed ability development of the girls differs from the boys. Among 8-year-old girls, a high level of development was seen in 50% of individuals in the clean zone and 11% in the polluted zone. Of the 9-year-old girls, a level above average was seen in 40% of the girls from the clean zone and 27% from the polluted zone. The average levels for the girls from the clean zone were: 10% for 8-year-olds, 12% for 9-year-olds and 10% for 10-year-olds. From the polluted zone the averages were: 46% for 8-year-olds, 80% for 9-year-olds and 29% for 10-year-olds. A low level of development was found in 90% of the girls from the clean zone. Among the 8- to 10-year-old children, most had an average or lower than average speed development ability.

The force development ability among the boys living in the clean zone was average or below average. The boys living in the zone of low doses of radiation had levels below average and low. Among the girls from both zones, the level of force development ability was below average or low. An average level of development was seen in 20–40% of the girls.

The level of development of endurance is given in table 7. The data presented in table 7 illustrates that by the level of development, 8-year-old children have a mean index in the clean zone (100%). Among the children living in the ecologically clean zone, the average level of endurance development ranges from 50 to 100%. Completely different levels of endurance development are observed in the children living in the zone with increased radiation. Below average levels are seen in 30–96% of the 8- to 10-year-old children and a low level of development is apparent in 7–70% of children, the level of the girls being higher than that of the boys.

Qualitative analysis of the physical development indices of the 8- to 10-year-old children living in conditions of increased radiation showed that, for most of the indices, the children have average, below average and low levels.

Qualitative changes are irregular both for individual indices characterizing physical state, and for the children as a whole. Further longitudinal studies of the development of children from polluted zones and their comparison with the development of children from clean zones are indispensable for the evaluation of the delayed effects of small doses of radiation during growth.

Summary and Conclusions

Comparative data on physical development and functional status of children before the Chernobyl accident (1985) and in 1990 were collected. The study provided the opportunity to evaluate differences in the physical condition of children living in the zone with increased radiation levels. The data show a progressive but irregular trend in growth and somatic development of youngsters aged 7–17 years. There is some evidence on the basis of these results of a stimulating action of small radiation doses. The effect is short-lived, approximately 2–3 years, and is followed by a sharp decline in growth rates. The physical state of children living in conditions of increased radiation generally reflects the age-related features, but there are definite peculiarities. Qualitative analysis of physical development indices of e.g. 8- to 10-year-old children living in conditions of increased radiation showed that the children have average, below average and low levels for most of the indices. Qualitative changes are irregular both as regards individual indices characterizing physical state, and the children in general. Deviations of different parameters vary in intensity and depend on a number of factors, including physical activity. These data quantify the delay of anticipated weight gains during these ages. Junior schoolchildren were classified as follows: average body height was recorded in 70% girls and 48% boys, average body weight in 44% girls and 30% boys. Clinical observations revealed various changes in the children. In particular, enlargement of the thyroid gland grade 1 and 2 was found in 82% of the girls and 65% of the boys. Lymphadenopathy was present in 63% girls and 21% boys. Dental caries was recorded in 79% girls and 72% boys, and cardiopathy in 26% girls and 21% boys.

The results of spirometry and PWC_{170} index characterize the level of physical work capacity for individuals. PWC_{170} declined with age from 7 to 9 years before increasing and then declining again at 10 years of age. PWC levels of all children were lower than expected. Studying the children over a long period of time showed an increased vegetative liability, general weakness, drowsiness and apathy.

The testing of motor development included a 20-meter run, throwing a tennis ball, throwing a weighted ball and a 6-min run. Each task was evaluated on a 5-point scale, 1 point for a low score and 5 points for a high score. The level of the development of running abilities of schoolchildren living in different ecological zones varied. Thus e.g. 9- to 10-year-old children living in ecologically clean zones had higher indices than children living in the zone of increased radiation, but in girls the situation was reversed. Eight- to 10-year-old boys in the ecologically clean zone also surpassed the boys living in the polluted zone on the 6-min running index. The 8- to 9-year-old boys from the clean zone had better results in pushing the weighted ball than boys of the same age living in the zone affected by small doses of radiation. The 8- to 10-year-old boys living in the ecologically clean zone also surpassed the boys living in the polluted zone on the 6-minute running index. The ability to hit a goal directly (deftness) is expressed by the results of tennis ball throwing; with respect to the developmental level of deftness differences are observed in the children from different ecological zones.

Comparison of the age and sex differences of children from different ecological zones showed, in most cases, a substantial superiority of children living in an ecologically clean zone. The unique environmental conditions due to increased radiation after the Chernobyl disaster calls for new approaches in the assessment of growth status and the physical training to facilitate functional improvement, without damaging the children's health.

References

1 Antonov VP: Radiatsionnaya obstanovka and yeyo sotsialno–psichologicheskiye aspekty. K Znaniye, 1987.
2 Glazyrina LD: Povyshaya soprotivlyayemost' radiatsyonnomu vozdejstviyu. Phyzicheskaya Kult shkolw 1991;10:46.
3 Dynnikova LA: Phizicheskiye uprazhneniya and onkologicheskiye zabolevaniya. Teoriya Praktika Phyzicheskoy Kult 1991;5:21.
4 Kullander S, Larsson B: Zhizn' posle Chernobylya. M: Energoatomizdat, 1991.
5 Nickberg II: Ioniziruyushchaya radiatsiya and zdorovye cheloveka. Kiev, Zdorovye, 1989, p 159.
6 Radiatsiya: Dozy, effekt, risk: Translation from English. M: Mir.
7 Holl G: Radiatsiya and zhyzn. M: Meditsina, 1989.

Dr. K. Kozlova, Vinnitsa State Pedagogic Institute,
K. Ostrovsky Street 32, 287100 Vinnitsa (Ukraine)

Growth and Motor Performances of Rural Senegalese Children

Eric Benefice

Chargé de Recherche, Laboratoire de Nutrition Tropicale,
Institut Français de Recherche Scientifique pour le
Développement en Coopération (ORSTOM), Montpellier, France

Introduction

In developing countries environmental constraints such as undernutrition, the high burden of infectious or parasitic diseases, bad living conditions including housing, economic precariousness, food crisis, lack of health or educational facilities must be taken into consideration when discussing growth and development of children. More than 20 years ago, it was shown that, in developing countries, difference in growth of preschool children associated with socioeconomic factors was many times greater than difference linked to ethnicity [1]. Delayed growth in terms of weight and stature are foremost indicators of health or nutritional disorders [2]. Moreover, environmental and nutritional factors appear to be more important during catch-up growth than genetic factors [3].

In Africa, the prevalence of malnutrition is especially high. While Senegal is not the most disadvantaged country (of the Sahelian belt) in this respect, malnutrition is widespread in rural areas. About 10% of 0- to 5-year-old children are wasted, that is, weight for stature is more than 2 standard deviations (SD) below the WHO/National Center for Health Statistics (NCHS) reference [4] and 26.5% are stunted, that is, stature-for-age children are 2 SD under the reference [5]. Data presented in this paper were collected in a rural area of Central Senegal; mild-to-moderate undernutrition is a major factor in the growth, physical fitness and motor characteristics of these children.

Malnutrition can interfere with the normal development of children in a variety of ways and at different times. During the fetal period and at the beginning of life, especially during the acceleration of brain growth and myelinization, malnutrition could directly affect cerebral development [6]. Later in life, opportunities for exercise, limb movements and exploratory behavior, which are of foremost importance for child development, may be decreased in order to balance energy requirements when intakes are low. This will change the child's attitudes and interactions with his caregivers [7]. Throughout the growing period, the persistence of undernutrition with reduced body size and muscle mass may influence motor development and physical fitness [8, 9]. This last issue will be the focus of this paper. The paper reports on the growth and performances of Senegalese children and examines the relationships between somatic and functional variables.

Methods

Selection of children

A total of 348 children, including 168 boys and 180 girls, were drawn from several health and fitness surveys undertaken between 1988 and 1994 in rural Senegal. Most children came from the central western part of the country known as the 'peanut basin' (14.45° north and 17.30° west). Fifty-nine children were from the district of Podor in the extreme north, in the bend of Senegal River. The age of the children at the time of the study ranged between 5 and 13 years. All were recruited after a home-by-home census in the villages and only children free from clinically detectable diseases were chosen. Less than 90 children in the study group regularly attended elementary school but no differences in anthropometry or motor performance were noted with the other children. Parents were poor Muslim farmers living at a subsistence level who grew peanuts and millet in the center, rice, sorghum and millet in the north. People from Central Senegal belonged to the Wolof ethnic group, and to the Tokolor ethnic group in the north. Slight but insignificant differences in anthropometric indices existed between the two ethnic groups. The basic diet of children consisted of rice and dry fish at midday and a gruel of sorghum at night. Energy and protein content of the diet was insufficient for more than one third of the families and deficiencies were common in retinol, riboflavin, zinc, calcium, folates and heminic iron [10, 11].

The aims and methods of the surveys were explained to parents, headmen and officials in the villages and oral consent was obtained. Examinations were conducted outdoors and in the presence of the mother or another member of the child's family.

Anthropometry

Children were weighed (kg) lightly clothed with an electronic scale precise to 100 g. Standing height (cm) was measured with a Harpenden® anthropometer. Arm circumferences (cm) were measured on the left side with a fiberglass ribbon. Subcutaneous triceps skinfold (mm) was recorded at the same level, in accordance with recommended techniques [12]. Arm muscle circumference (cm) was calculated as [13]: $MUAC = AC - \Pi \times TSF$.

Cardiorespiratory fitness

In younger children (5–6 years of age) cardiorespiratory adaptation to effort was estimated after a submaximal step test proposed by Čermák et al. [14] and modified by Pařízková [15] in preschool children. After a preliminary rest period of 3 min in the sitting position, children had to climb up and down a two step ladder with rungs of 23 cm in height. They stepped for a 5-min period at a rhythm of 30 steps/min. At the end of the test they sat and rested for 5 min. In older children (≥ 7 years of age) a step test with 3 benches of different heights (17, 23 and 30 cm) were used. Children rested for 3 min and then climbed up and down the steps for 3 min at each bench height, at a rhythm of 30 steps/min. This allowed a gradual increase of effort. They then sat and rested for 5 min. For the duration of the testing session, heart rate frequency (beats per minute, bpm) was recorded every 5 s using a Sport tester monitor (Polar Electro Oy®).

Motor performances

Measures of performance included a 20-meter dash in <6-year-old children and a 33-meter dash in ≤ 6 year-old children (expressed as speed: m/s), a tennis ball throw for distance in <6-year-old children and a soft ball throw in ≥ 6-year-old children, hand grip strength was estimated by squeezing a rubber bulb connected to a manometer Martin®, and a standing long jump. Children performed 3 trials of jump, throw and hand grip tests following practice sessions the day before.

Analysis

Statistical analysis was performed using the routines of the BMDP® statistical software. Reliability of the measures was estimated by measuring a subsample of 40 children twice with a 1-day interval. Test-retest correlation coefficients were moderate for dash (0.67), jump (0.73) and grip strength (0.71), and high for the throw (0.93). No gender difference in reliability was observed.

Results

Figure 1 shows the weight and stature curves by age for boys (fig. 1a) and girls (fig. 1b). They are compared to the median and 5th percentile of the NCHS reference data [4]. Senegalese boys display a marked retardation compared with the reference, between 10 and 12 years of age their growth slows down. This trend is less pronounced in the case of girls. Girls older than 8 years reach significantly higher values than boys in weight but not in stature.

After classifying children in three age groups, 4–6.9 years (preschool children), 7–10.5 years (preadolescents), ≥ 10.5 years (beginning of adolescence), mean values for triceps skinfold, arm circumference and arm muscle circumference were compared with medians of the National Health and Nutrition Survey I [16] taken as reference (fig. 2). Values for Senegalese children are always inferior. For example, triceps skinfold is about one half, and arm circumference and arm muscle circumference are 20–25% lower than the refer-

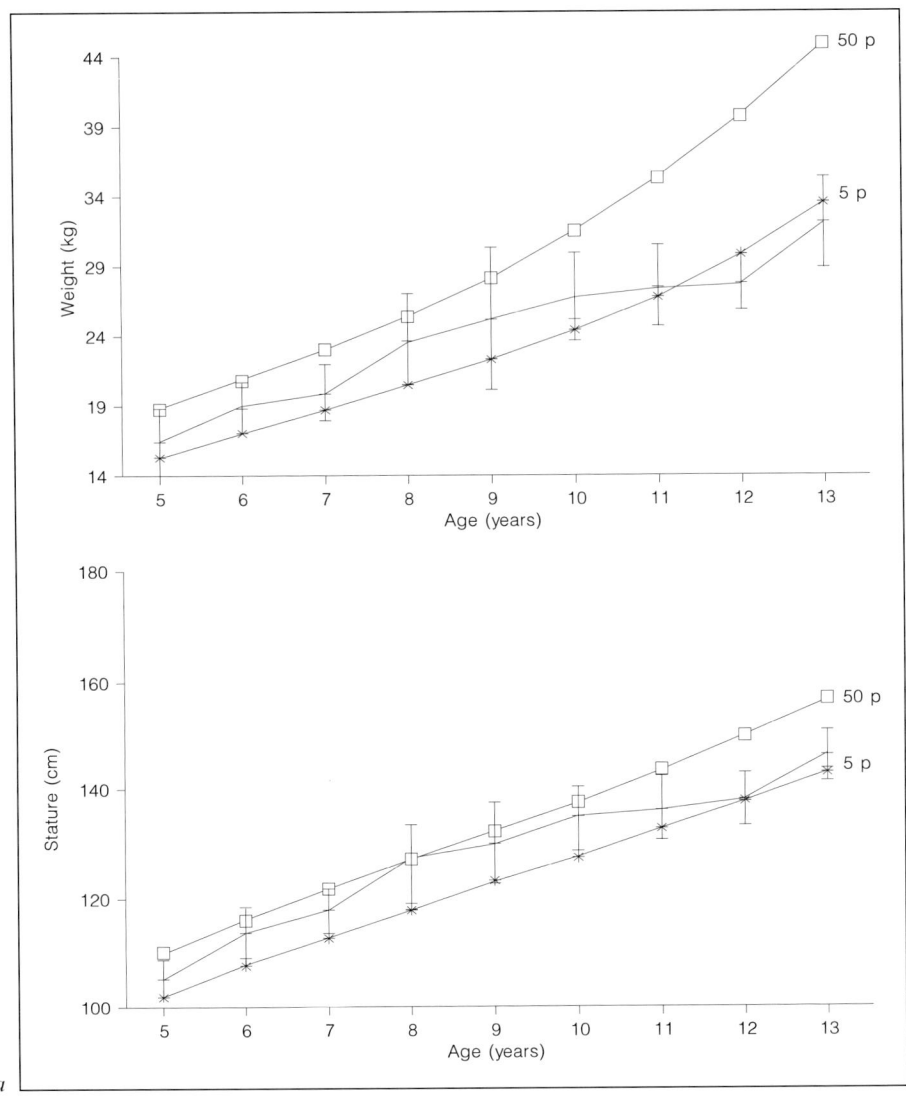

Fig. 1. Weight and stature of boys (*a*) and girls (*b*) (mean, SD) relative to the 5th and 50th percentiles of US reference data.

ence. In addition, girls have consistently higher values (p < 0.001) than boys for these three indices.

Body mass index (BMI = weight/stature^2) is a common indicator of body composition and fatness for populations. Figure 3 shows the BMI by age of Senegalese children plotted against a population of healthy French children

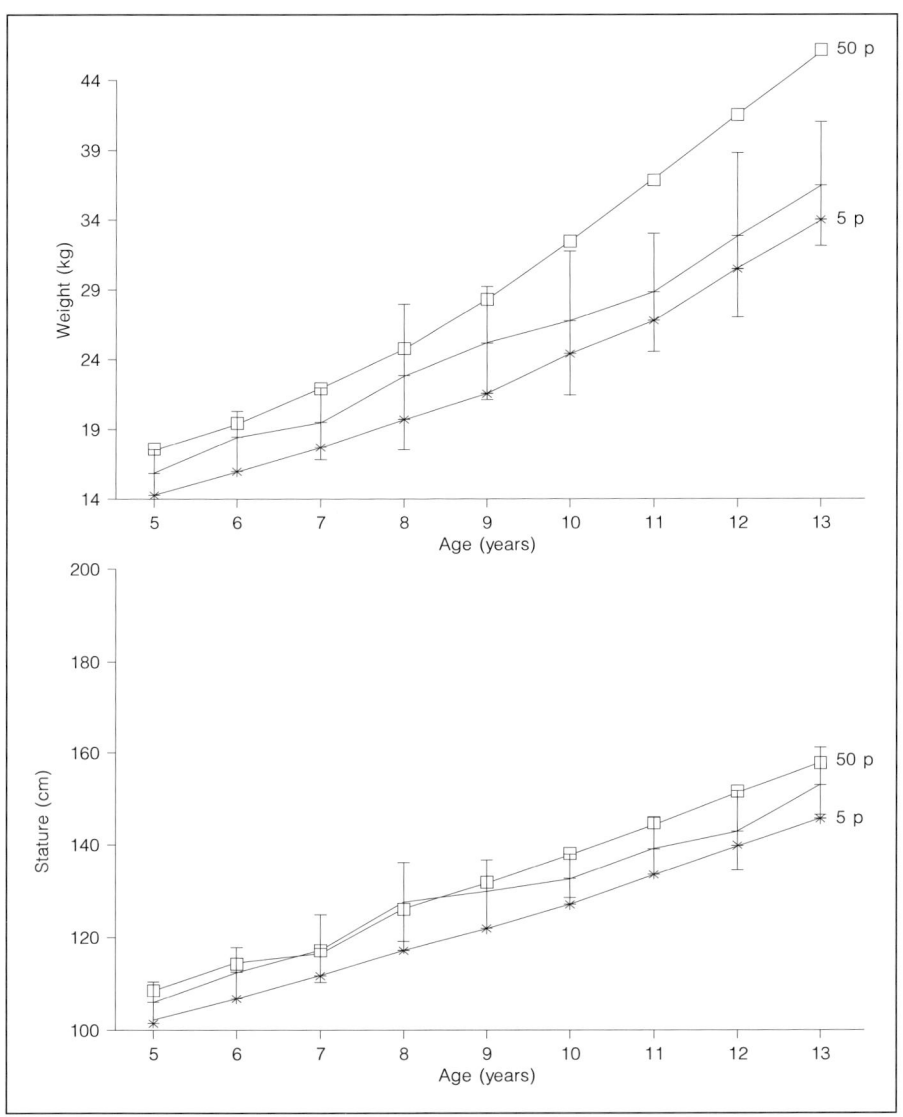

b

[17]. Senegalese children were clearly below the mean values recorded for the French population. BMI for girls tends to increase at 10 years of age, while it levels off in the case of boys.

Means and standard deviations for motor tasks are shown in table 1. In contrast with anthropometric indices, boys achieve better performances than

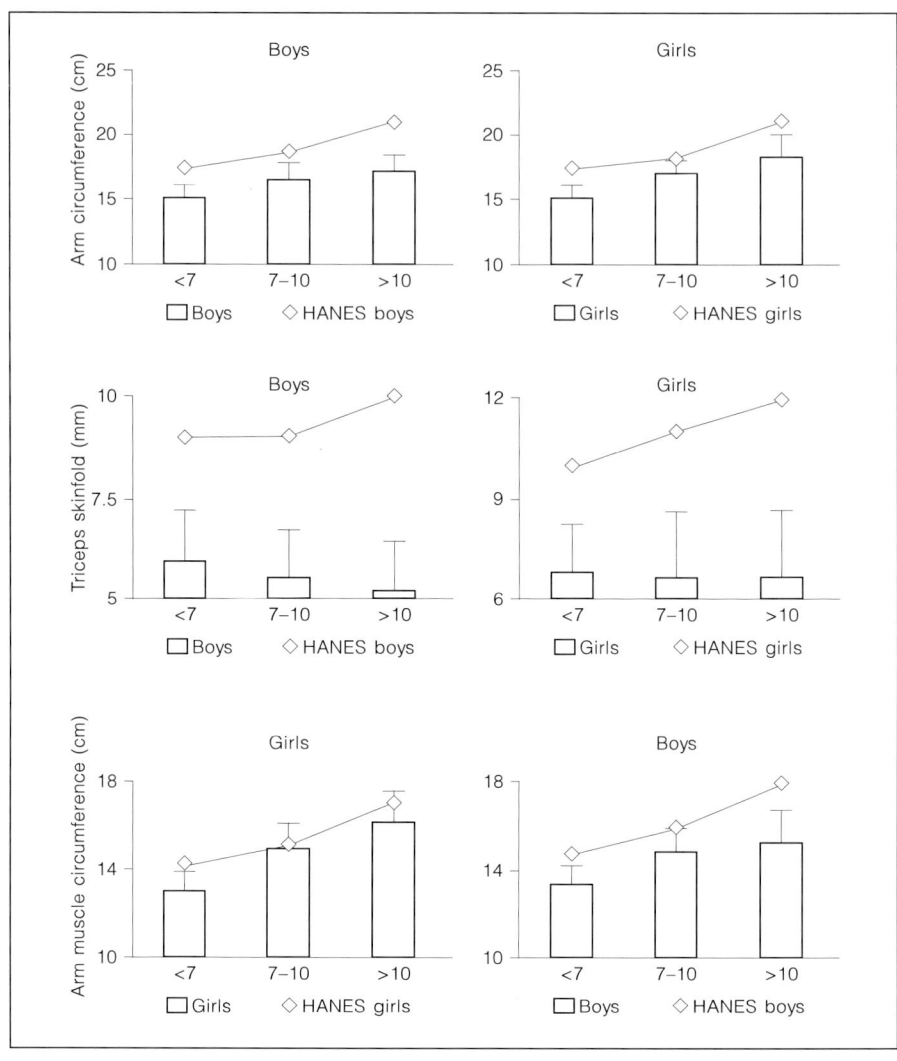

Fig. 2. Arm circumference, triceps skinfold, and arm muscle circumference of Senegalese boys and girls (mean, SD) relative to the median of US reference data (HANES I).

girls in speed, jump and throw. However, results for grip strength are more variable.

Figure 4 represents the heart rate (HR) changes during exercise. Senegalese preschool children are compared with healthy Czech children of the same age (fig. 4a). During the step test at rest and during recovery, HRs are significantly

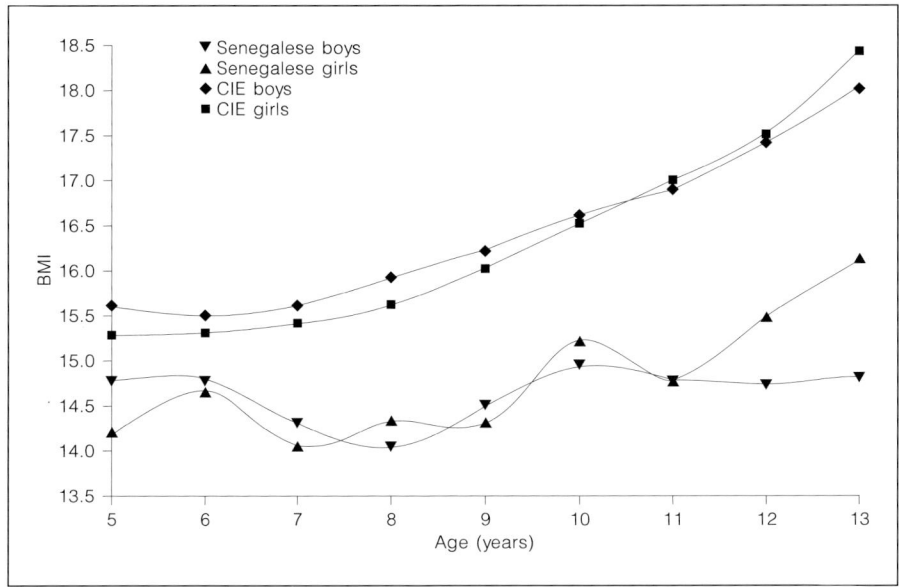

Fig. 3. BMI of Senegalese children (mean, SD) relative to the mean of healthy French children.

lower in boys than in girls (p<0.001). Senegalese children had higher HR during exercise and recovery than Czech children. Senegalese girls had the higher HR at rest, during exercise and recovery than all the other children. Changes in HR of older children during the step test appear in figure 4b. Boys achieved significantly lower values than girls during exercise and recovery. In young as well as in older children, the maximum reduction in HR occurred during the 1st min of recovery.

Sex-specific relationships between motor performances and growth are shown in table 2. The independent variables used in the model are age, stature, weight and BMI. This model is a significant predictor of performances in both sexes. However, the percent of variance explained is modest for speed, where no variable has a significant effect, and for hand grip strength in boys. BMI has a significant effect in jump and hand grip strength in both sexes, and in speed performance of boys. Regression coefficients between body mass and performances are always negative.

To further explore relationships between motor performance and body composition, comparisons were done in the upper and lower quartile of BMI of the three age groups. To exclude the sex effect, variables were standardized

Table 1. Motor performance (means and SD) of Senegalese children

Age years	n	Speed m/s	Jump m	Throw m	Grip strength kPa
Boys					
5	15	3.2	0.74	4.6	48.6
		0.4	0.19	1.0	12.7
6	24	3.6	0.94	7.9	64.6
		0.4	0.20	2.0	16.6
7	24	3.8	1.03	8.4	78.3
		0.5	0.20	2.0	19.6
8	18	3.9	1.25	12.4	88.9
		0.4	0.21	3.2	22.1
9	7	4.2	1.33	14.2	98.1
		0.3	0.19	3.6	26.4
10	23	4.3	1.37	15.5	108.1
		0.3	0.20	4.0	34.0
11	27	4.4	1.41	15.3	115.3
		0.3	0.19	2.5	22.7
12	15	4.5	1.42	17.2	106.9
		0.4	0.16	3.9	28.0
13	15	4.5	1.52	17.7	107.6
		0.4	0.18	3.4	27.0
Girls					
5	23	3.3	0.75	4.2	49.7
		0.4	0.22	1.5	10.3
6	25	3.3	0.88	5.9	66.1
		0.5	0.20	2.1	13.5
7	18	3.3	0.97	7.0	81.4
		0.5	0.22	2.2	18.4
8	13	3.5	1.09	8.3	75.6
		0.4	0.18	3.2	21.1
9	25	3.9	1.19	10.8	90.4
		0.4	0.16	2.6	16.8
10	18	3.9	1.33	11.1	96.6
		0.5	0.23	2.6	29.3
11	30	4.0	1.36	12.5	108.4
		0.5	0.21	2.6	27.2
12	22	4.5	1.43	14.7	117.7
		0.5	0.17	4.1	32.0
13	6	4.4	1.37	14.7	112.6
		0.9	0.24	3.8	23.6
2-way analysis of variance					
F age		31.2	58.1	76.8	27.4
p		<0.001	<0.001	<0.001	<0.001
F sex		26.9	8.8	64.4	29.4
p		<0.001	<0.001	<0.001	<0.001

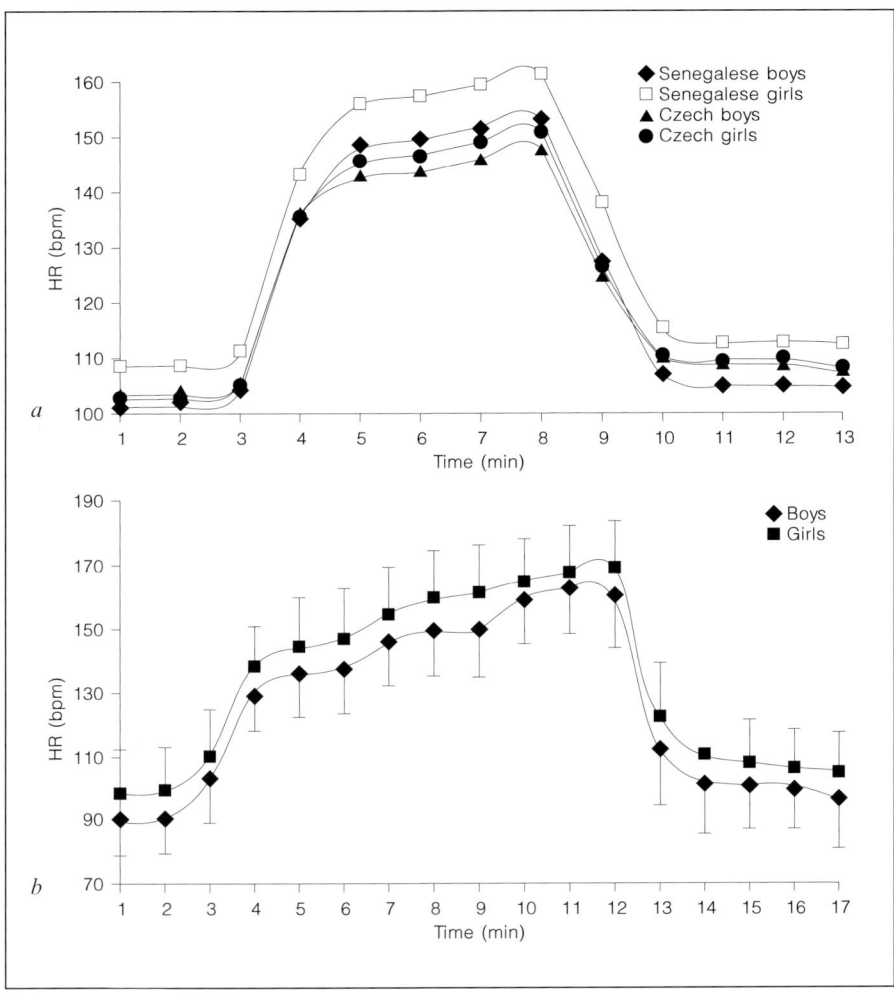

Fig. 4. HR during step test in Senegalese preschool children compared with Czech children (*a*) and in Senegalese children ≥7 years of age (*b*; mean ±95% confidence interval).

in each age group. A standardized variable is equal to $(X_{observed} - X_{group})/SD$ where $X_{observed}$ is the observed value and X_{group} the group mean. Under these conditions, there are no significant differences between BMI groups among younger children, while children with higher BMI tended to perform better. Figure 5 indicates that in the two other age groups, all differences are significant; children in the upper quartile of BMI are always superior to children in the lower quartile.

Table 2. Regression of motor performances and strength on age, stature, BMI and weight in Senegalese children

Dependent variable	Independent variables	Regression coefficient	t	p
Boys (n=168)				
Speed	age	0.0035	1.73	NS
	stature	0.07	3.35	<0.001
	BMI	0.28	2.90	<0.02
	weight	−0.12	2.23	<0.02
	R^2	0.61		
	F	66.0		
Jump	age	0.0015	1.46	NS
	stature	0.031	2.98	<0.003
	MBI	0.10	2.24	<0.02
	weight	−0.044	1.59	NS
	R^2	0.66		
	F	82.0		
Throw	age	0.036	2.35	<0.02
	ature	0.25	1.57	NS
	BMI	0.62	0.85	NS
	weight	−0.038	0.09	NS
	R^2	0.72		
	F	105.6		
Grip strength	age	0.026	0.20	NS
	stature	2.45	1.85	<0.06
	BMI	10.72	1.78	NS
	weight	−2.57	0.73	NS
	R^2	0.50		
	F	41.8		

Discussion

Senegalese children displayed obvious backwardness in somatic growth compared with an international reference. They also appear to have less subcutaneous fat and total fatness than American or European children. In both sexes, triceps skinfold thickness are at or below the 5th percentile of the National Health and Nutrition Survey I [16]. An obvious reason is an inadequate coverage of energy and nutrient requirements. Other unfavorable conditions such as transmissible diseases and poor housing must also be

Table 2 (continued)

Dependent variable	Independent variables	Regression coefficient	t	p
Girls (n=180)				
Speed	age	0.000	0.25	NS
	stature	0.031	1.40	NS
	BMI	0.044	0.43	NS
	weight	−0.01	0.31	NS
	R^2	0.41		
	F	30.5		
Jump	age	0.002	2.33	<0.02
	stature	0.029	3.40	<0.008
	BMI	0.11	2.75	<0.006
	weight	−0.05	2.43	<0.01
	R^2	0.63		
	F	74.6		
Throw	age	0.029	2.12	<0.03
	stature	0.287	2.67	<0.008
	BMI	0.88	1.79	NS
	weight	−0.28	1.08	NS
	R^2	0.72		
	F	116.1		
Grip strength	age	0.31	2.56	<0.01
	stature	2.32	2.44	<0.01
	BMI	13.58	3.12	<0.002
	weight	−4.40	1.94	<0.05
	R^2	0.56		
	F	55.82		

considered. In Africa, these conditions are generally worse in rural than in urban settings [18]. During puberty, many changes in body size and composition occur which results in a progressive increase in BMI [17]. Older children studied, especially boys, do not exhibit such an increase which suggests a delay in the adolescent growth spurt. This is consistent with other studies from Africa [19] and with recent research from a neighboring area in Senegal which reports a 3-year delay in age at menarche [21]. Such delays in growth and maturation at adolescence could also be linked to undernutrition [20].

Motor performances of Senegalese children would also appear to be lower than those of healthy children. Senegalese children perform poorly compared to children from the Czech Republic for preschool ages [15] or from the USA for older children [22].

During the step test, girls displayed higher HR than boys and boys had lower HR at rest and during recovery; this suggests less HR per unit of load to be carried up and down and thus a better cardiac efficiency among boys. This difference is consistent with other data from literature [23–25].

Body dimensions are an important determinant of performance in undernourished children [8]. In this study, stature and body mass have a significant effect on performances independently of the age effect. This suggests that a part of the variance in performances could be explained by stature and weight within the same age group. Performances are positively related to stature but negatively to weight. Small children are disadvantaged with regard to tall children of the same age. A negative relationship between weight and performance is not surprising especially in tasks where the body is projected or with rapid movement such as dash or throw; an excessive weight may increase the load to be carried [26].

However, lean children performed poorly compared with bigger children as it is illustrated by comparing performances in the upper and lower quartile of BMI. Differences were not significant for preschool children, possibly as in young children motor patterns are not fully established and factors such as motivation, apprehension, and previous experience may play a relatively more important role than in older children. A higher BMI is indicative of higher fat-free mass and fat mass per unit of stature. In mild to moderately undernourished children, fatness may thus be considered as an indicator of larger body size and better nutritional status, consistent with previous research [27].

Senegalese children in this study displayed some degree of growth retardation which may be responsible for their poor motor performances. Changes in body composition with age are also significant predictors of motor performances. It must be emphasized that better nutritional status associated with better performance is an important issue for the agricultural development of nonmechanised societies.

Summary and Conclusions

Anthropometric measurements (height, weight, skinfolds), motor performance (dash, standing long jump, throw, hand grip strength), and a submaximal step test were performed in 348 Senegalese children (168 boys and 180

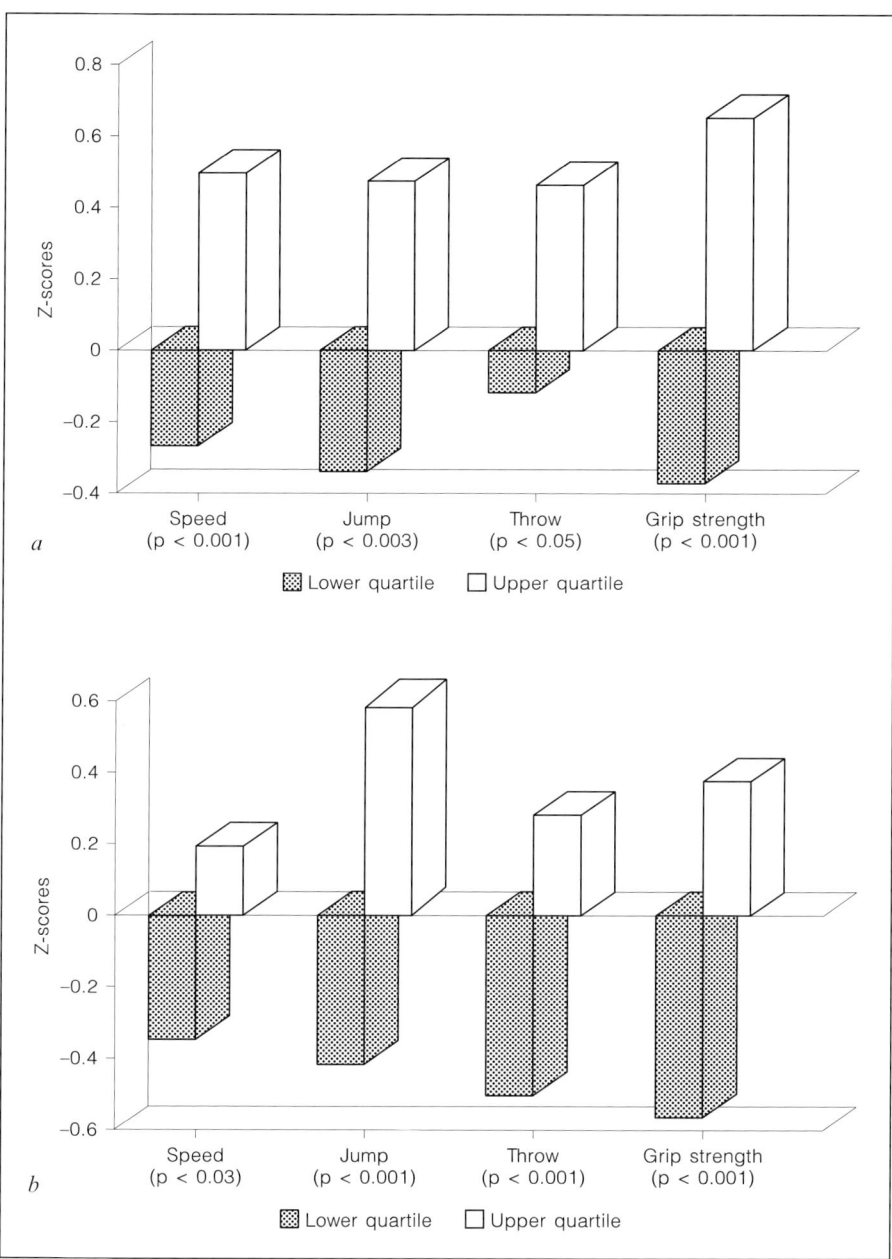

Fig. 5. Motor performance (z-scores) of Senegalese children aged 6–10 years (*a*) and > 10 years (*b*) in the lower and upper quartiles of BMI.

girls) between 5 and 13 years of age. Girls tended to have higher anthropometric values than boys, but boys were superior in motor tasks and presented a better cardiorespiratory response to exercise. Children were delayed in growth compared with the WHO/NCHS reference data and could be considered as mild-to-moderately undernourished. Variance in motor performance was partly explained by body dimensions. In children older than 7 years, those with high BMI performed better in all tasks than those with low BMI. Functional consequences of chronic malnutrition are an important issue in rural African society where subsistence depends on physical work.

References

1 Habicht JP, Martorell R, Yarrough C, Malina RM, Klein RE: Height and weight standards for preschool children. How relevant are ethnic differences in growth potential. Lancet 1974;i:611–615.
2 Tanner JM: Growth as a monitor of nutritional status. Proc Nutr Soc 1976;35:315–322.
3 Lewinter-Suskind L, Fuchs GJ, Kaewkantha S, Suskind RM: Long-term growth potential of previously malnourished children; in Suskind RM, Lewinter-Suskind L (eds): The Malnourished Child. Nestlé Nurition Workshop Series. New York, Raven Press, 1990, vol 19, pp 383–393.
4 World Health Organization: Measuring Change in Nutritional Status. Geneva, World Health Organization, 1983.
5 Ndiaye S, Diouf PD, Ayad M: Enquête Démographique et de Santé (EDS-II). Dakar, Ministère du Plan, 1994.
6 Dobbing J, Sands J: Quantitative growth and development of human brain. Arch Dis Child 1973; 48:757–767.
7 Politt E: A critical view of three decades of research on the effects of chronic energy malnutrition and behavioural development; in Schurch B, Scrimshaw N (eds): Chronic Energy Deficiency: Consequenses and Related Issues. IDECG Meeting August 1987. Lausanne, Nestlé Foundation, 1987, pp 77–93.
8 Malina RM: Physical activity and motor development/performance in population nutritionally at risk; in Pollitt E, Amante P (eds): Energy Intake and Activity. New York, Liss, 1984, pp 285–302.
9 Spurr GB: Body size, physical work capacity, and productivity in hard work: Is bigger better?; in Waterlow JC (ed): Linear Growth Retardation in Less Developed Countries. New York, Raven Press, 1988, pp 215–243.
10 Chevassus-Agnès S, Ndiaye AM: Enquêtes de consommation alimentaire de l'ORANA de 1977 à 1979: Méthodologie et résultats; in Etat Nutritionnel de la Population Rurale de Sahel. Ottawa, CRDI, 1981, pp 57–66.
11 Benefice E, Simondon K: Agricultural development and nutrition among rural populations: A case study of the middle valley in Senegal. Ecol Food Nutr 1993;31:45–66.
12 Weiner JS, Lourie JA: Practical Human Biology. London, Academic Press, 1981.
13 Gurney J, Jelliffe DB: Arm anthropometry in nutritional assessment: Nomogram for rapid calculation of muscle circumference and cross-sectional muscle and fat areas. Am J Clin Nutr 1973;26:912–915.
14 Čermák J, Čermaková J, Zudova Z, Cerma M, Tuma S: Die Unterschiede in der Funktionstüchtigkeit des Kreislaufsystems von Schülern der Experimental-Schwimmklassen im Vergleich mit gleichalten, keinen Sport treibenden Schülern. Schweiz Z Sportmed 1969;1:9–19.
15 Pařízková J: Nutrition, Physical Activity, and Health in Early Life. New York, CRC Press, 1996.
16 Frisancho AR: New norms for upper limb fat and muscle areas for assessment of nutritional status. Am J Clin Nutr 1981;34:2540–2545.
17 Rolland-Cachera MF, Cole TJ, Sempé M, Tichet J, Rossignol C, Charraud A: Body mass index variations: Centiles from birth to 87 years. Eur J Clin Nutr 1991;45:13–21.

18 Corlett JT, Woollard E: Growth patterns of rural children in the region of Botswana. Ann Hum Biol 1988;15:153–159.
19 Cameron N, Kgamphe JS: The growth of South African rural black children. S Afr Med J 1993; 83:184–190.
20 Kulin HE, Bwibo N, Mutie D, Santner SJ: The effect of chronic childhood malnutrition on pubertal growth and development. Am J Clin Nutr 1982;36:527–536.
21 Simondon KB, Simon I, Simondon F: Nutritional status and age at menarche of Senegalese adolescents. Ann Hum Biol 1997;24:521–532.
22 Malina RM, Roche AF: Manual of Physical Status and Performance in Childhood. New York, Plenum Press, 1983, vol 2: Physical Performance.
23 Benefice E: Growth and motor performance of healthy Senegalese preschool children. Am J Hum Biol 1992;4:717–728.
24 Benefice E: Physical activity, cardiorespiratory fitness, motor performance, and growth of Senegalese pre-adolescents. Am J Hum Biol 1993;5:653–667.
25 Braden DS, Strong WB: Cardiovascular responses to exercise in childhood. Am J Dis Child 1990; 114:1255–1260.
26 Malina RM: Anthropometry, strength and motor fitness; in Ulijaszek SJ, Mascie-Taylor CGN (eds): Anthropometry: The Individual and the Population. Cambridge, Cambridge University Press, 1994, pp 160–177.
27 Malina RM, Little BB: Body composition, strength, and motor performance in undernourished boys; in Binkhorst RA, Kemper HCG, Saris WHM (eds): Children and Exercise. Champaign, Human Kinetics, 1985, vol 4, pp 293–300.

Eric Benefice, Laboratoire de Nutrition Tropicale, ORSTOM,
911 av Agropolis, BP 5045, F–34032 Montpellier (France)

Cardiorespiratory Fitness and Body Composition in Indian Children of 10–16 Years

G.L. Khanna, P. Majumdar, M. Saha, M. Mandal

Faculty of Sports Sciences, Sports Authority of India, Netaji Subhas Southern Centre, Bangalore, India

Introduction

The health and fitness of an individual during childhood and adolescence has a bearing on both physical growth and physical work capacity. A clear understanding of health status during the growth and development years has numerous potential benefits for education and health care systems. One might expect improvement in society's ability to better serve the needs of an individual child during these formative years. The development of age-specific training programs in sports have contributed to the need to know how the working capacity and exercise responses of the human body are affected during the growth period.

Fitness is best measured by maximum aerobic capacity of the individual and represents the limit of the organism's ability to utilize atmospheric oxygen for cellular energetics. This capacity presents an overall picture of the functional integration of the heart, lungs, circulation of blood and the active muscles in aerobic work [1–3]. The developed European and North American countries have provided valuable information on the physiological aspects during the growing years [3–7]. In the Asian region, Japan, Malaysia and China are the leading countries in the study of physiological responses to exercise in children using ergometry [8–10]. However, the main focus in Asian countries had been on the evaluation of cardiorespiratory responses in sportspersons.

Body composition also changes during growth and with ageing in relation to health, nutrition and physical activity. Pařízková [11] observed that the magnitude of change in body composition varies with the intensity and duration of physical activity among boys. Physique and body composition have an important role in the performance of various physical activities. Body fat percentages of children in different countries have been reported by a number of scientists [3, 7, 11, 12] but studies on Indian children are scanty [13, 14]. Fry et al. [15] reported on the importance of economic status on body composition status. Children from high socioeconomic groups possessed more subcutaneous fat than middle and low socioeconomic groups. Generally, previous research has indicated that in primitive communities the populations are leaner compared to counterparts in developed countries. In India, some attempts have been made to study the morphological and physiological aspects of the developing child [13, 14].

There is a growing interest in the selection and training of young athletes to facilitate maximal performance in adulthood. Whilst the growth and maturity characteristics of children active in sports may be related to systematic training from an early age [16], the contribution of physical activity and growth to a change in the fitness level is uncertain. There is a need to evaluate the cardiopulmonary responses of children and adolescents in the 10- to 16-year age group during graded ergometry under aerobic and anaerobic conditions. The monitoring of growth and development from a morphological and physiological point of view has been fragmentary and has not provided a concise and comprehensive picture in Indian children.

Materials and Methods

The present investigation is based on a cross-sectional analysis of 777 children involved in training for high level sports performance and a further 209 schoolchildren of 10–16 years of age. Children comprising the training group were selected by the coaches and scientists on the basis of their performance and motor qualities from all over India. The untrained reference group was composed of children from various schools. The age of subjects was attained verbally and was confirmed from records and converted into decimal age. Subjects were weighed with a minimum of clothing (shorts) on a weighing machine with an accuracy of 10 g. Stature was measured with a stadiometer to an accuracy of 0.1 cm.

Body fat was calculated indirectly from skinfold thickness and based on the widely accepted formulae of Pařízková and Roth [17]. Skinfolds were measured using a Harpenden skinfold caliper at four sites, biceps, triceps, subscapular and suprailiac. Body fat was calculated from body density using the formula of Siri [18].

Cycle ergometry was employed for the evaluation of cardiopulmonary response as most Indian School children are familiar with cycling as a modality of physical activity. A graded protocol of exercise starting with a work load of 1 W/kg of body weight and increased by 0.5 W/kg thereafter till exhaustion, until a plateau of VO_2 was attained or the respiratory quotient increased beyond 1.1 [13] or the subject was unable to continue pedalling at the required pace. Oxygen consumption (VO_2), carbon dioxide production, ventilation (VE), heart rate and oxygen pulse were recorded every 30 s on a computerized EOS Sprint (Jaeger, Germany). During the recovery phase, the physiological variables were monitored until the oxygen consumption returned to the normal resting level. Oxygen debt was calculated by the standard method described by Fox et al. [19].

Table 1. Morphological characteristics of trained (Trd) and untrained (Utrd) Indian children of 10–16 years of age

Age group years	Weight, kg		Height, cm		Body fat, %		LBM, kg	
	Utrd	Trd	Utrd	Trd	Utrd	Trd	Utrd	Trd
10	28.10 ±5.91	31.73 ±3.84**	133.26 ±5.18	144.06 ±5.69**	16.14 ±3.75	13.31 ±3.07**	24.20 ±3.52	27.46 ±3.13
11	28.36 ±3.61	35.16 ±5.52**	135.82 ±4.82	148.25 ±8.32**	13.94 ±3.13	13.28 ±3.13 (NS)	24.30 ±2.52	30.34 ±4.47**
12	31.80 ±3.83	38.80 ±5.84**	142.66 ±7.35	153.18 ±7.74**	13.91 ±2.81	13.52 ±2.75 (NS)	27.00 ±3.55	33.45 ±4.95**
13	37.80 ±6.87	41.80 ±6.46**	150.21 ±8.23	156.62 ±8.04**	14.51 ±3.81	13.53 ±2.71 (NS)	31.09 ±5.77	36.09 ±5.41**
14	44.58 ±6.96	45.67 ±7.06 (NS)	158.76 ±7.58	161.13 ±7.56 (NS)	13.77 ±3.18	12.89 ±2.28 (NS)	39.10 ±5.58	39.60 ±5.92 (NS)
15	45.51 ±6.55	49.68 ±5.97**	162.66 ±7.68	165.23 ±6.97 (NS)	14.35 ±3.10	13.56 ±2.48 (NS)	38.92 ±5.08	42.79 ±4.96**
16	51.76 ±6.26	53.30 ±7.87 (NS)	167.85 ±6.83	166.84 ±8.99 (NS)	15.40 ±2.87	14.48 ±2.85 (NS)	43.60 ±5.44	45.30 ±6.76 (NS)

Values represent mean ± SD. LBM = Lean body mass; NS = nonsignificant.

Results

Morphological characteristics of the subjects are presented in table 1. The weight of untrained Indian children varied from a mean of 28.1 kg at 10 years to 51.76 kg at 16 years whereas the trained children had significantly higher weights ($p < 0.01$) except at the age of 14 and 16 years. The maximum gain in weight was observed from 13 to 14 years in the untrained group (approximately 6.7 years), whereas in trained boys the maximum gain of 4.0 kg was observed in the 14–15 years of age group. The higher weight in the trained group may be due to selection, better nutrition and physical activity.

The body fat percent was not significantly different except at 10 years of age. This result revealed that growth, development and training may not significantly alter the body composition of boys. Lean body mass in the untrained group increased from a mean of 24.2 kg at 10 years to 43.6 kg at 16 years of age, whereas the trained group had significantly higher values in all the corresponding age groups except the 14- and 16-year age groups.

Table 2. Physiological characteristics of trained (Trd) and untrained (Utrd) Indian children of 10–16 years of age

Age group years	VO_{2max}, l/min		VO_{2max}, ml/kg/min		V_{Emax}, l/min		O_2 debt, l		O_2 pulse, m/beat		Maximum HR, bpm	
	Utrd	Trd	Utrd	Trd	Utrd	Trd	Utrd	Trd	Utrd	Trd	Utrd	Trd
10	1.10 ±0.20	1.65 ±0.29**	41.3 ±7.4	51.8 ±6.9**	45.68 ±9.38	61.99 ±14.1**	1.21 ±0.49	1.38 ±0.48 (NS)	5.81 ±0.94	8.40 ±1.57**	200.1 ±7.1	196.7 ±9.9 (NS)
11	1.18 ±0.22	1.82 ±0.33**	41.8 ±8.0	52.2 ±6.1**	50.30 ±11.4	67.90 ±15.4**	1.38 ±0.38	1.53 ±0.51 (NS)	5.87 ±1.08	9.30 ±1.71**	198.2 ±6.7	195.8 ±7.7 (NS)
12	1.35 ±0.30	2.13 ±0.38**	43.4 ±8.8	55.1 ±6.2**	54.85 ±12.4	78.10 ±15.0**	1.53 ±0.56	1.87 ±0.78*	6.84 ±1.53	10.86 ±1.90**	197.8 ±8.0	196.8 ±8.1 (NS)
13	1.66 ±0.36	2.38 ±0.44**	49.4 ±8.5	56.6 ±6.0**	64.48 ±12.2	88.62 ±17.1**	2.25 ±0.71	2.17 ±0.93 (NS)	9.71 ±2.12	11.86 ±2.24**	192.3 ±9.95	199.1 ±8.1**
14	2.16 ±0.46	2.69 ±0.49**	47.0 ±7.9	59.1 ±5.8**	74.74 ±13.9	98.52 ±18.8**	2.75 ±0.72	2.71 ±1.08 (NS)	11.41 ±2.56	13.61 ±2.54**	193.3 ±8.7	198.4 ±7.7**
15	2.00 ±0.46	2.90 ±0.45**	44.0 ±7.5	58.4 ±5.9**	73.60 ±11.4	105.6 ±19.9**	2.54 ±0.86	3.20 ±1.13**	10.96 ±2.75	14.61 ±2.30**	196.6 ±7.62	198.9 ±8.5**
16	2.45 ±0.47	3.10 ±0.57**	47.3 ±6.5	58.9 ±7.4**	82.97 ±16.2	115.6 ±22.8**	3.00 ±0.93	3.78 ±1.53**	12.78 ±3.04	15.64 ±2.76**	189.2 ±11.6	196.6 ±9.0**

Values represent mean ±SD. HR = Heart rate; NS = nonsignificant.

The physiological characteristics of subjects are presented in table 2. In the untrained group, the mean value of VO_{2max} was 1.11 liters/min at the age of 10 years and increased to 2.45 liters/min at the age of 16 years. In the trained group, both VO_{2max} and relative VO_{2max} were significantly higher ($p > 0.01$) at all ages. The rate of increment in VO_{2max} in both groups was very similar, 0.23 and 0.24 liters/min/year, respectively. The largest increment was observed from 12 to 13 years in the untrained group and from 15 to 16 years in the trained group. The highest relative VO_{2max} was observed at the age of 13 years in the untrained group (49.4 ml/kg/min) and 14 years in the trained group (59.4 ml/kg/min).

In the untrained children, the mean value of V_{Emax} was 45.68 liters/min at the age of 10 years and increased to 82.97 liters/min at the age of 16 years. In contrast, the V_{Emax} of the trained group was 61.99 liters/min at the age of 10 years and increased to 115.6 liters/min at the age of 16 years. Values for the trained group were significantly higher in each age group. The rate of increment in V_{Emax} in the untrained group was 6.28 compared with 8.94 liters/min/year in the trained group. The largest annual increment for the untrained was between 13 and 14 years and between 15 and 16 years in the trained group.

The mean maximum heart rate of untrained children ranged from a high of 200.1 to 186.6 bpm at 16 years of age. The maximum heart rate in the trained group did not change considerably. Differences in group means were significant in the 13- to 16-year age groups.

Discussion

Weight

The body weight of trained children in the present study was comparatively higher than that of untrained Indian children [20] and consistent with earlier investigations [21, 22]. This result is indicative of the positive training effect on muscle mass. However, comparisons between trained Indian children and corresponding age groups in developed countries indicate that the Indians are lighter than American, German, Hungarian and Dutch counterparts (fig.1) [23–26]. In contrast, Indian children were heavier than Tibetan and Nykyugan children [21]. Differences may be attributed to differences in socioeconomic status, nutrition and genetics.

Height

Interestingly, the trained Indian children were taller when compared with Dutch [26], German [24] and American [22] children at 10–11 years of age. Whilst still comparable at 12–13 years, international counterparts were taller

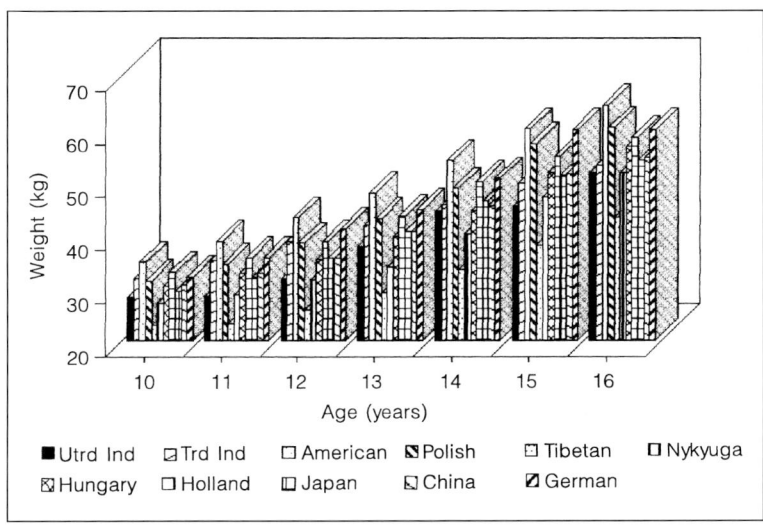

Fig. 1. Comparison of body weight of Indian children with their international counterparts. Utrd = Untrained; Trd = trained; Ind = Indian.

at all subsequent ages (fig. 2). Peak height velocity was also lower than in other populations.

Body Fat

Whilst there is no general agreement on the ideal amount of body fat in children, Shephard [3] has suggested the percentage should not exceed 17%. Children in both groups displayed a percent body fat lower than 17% with the trained group lower than the untrained but not significantly so. Rode and Shephard [27] explained that a high degree of physical activity may lead to smaller skinfold totals thereby improving heat dissipation. Body fat percentages for Indian trained and untrained children are also lower than for American, Norwegian and Canadian counterparts [13] (fig. 3). For example, Avlontiou [28] reported 17.2% body fat in trained swimmers of 12–13 years. Differences in body fat have been ascribed to the economic status [15], standard of living [27] and nutritional habits [29]. Stability of body fat with growth has also been reported by other scientists [7, 11, 31].

Aerobic Capacity

Aerobic capacity is largely determined by maximum cardiac output and A–VO$_2$ difference which in turn is dependent on stroke volume and heart rate. Aerobic exercise in adults improves the transport of oxygen by improved

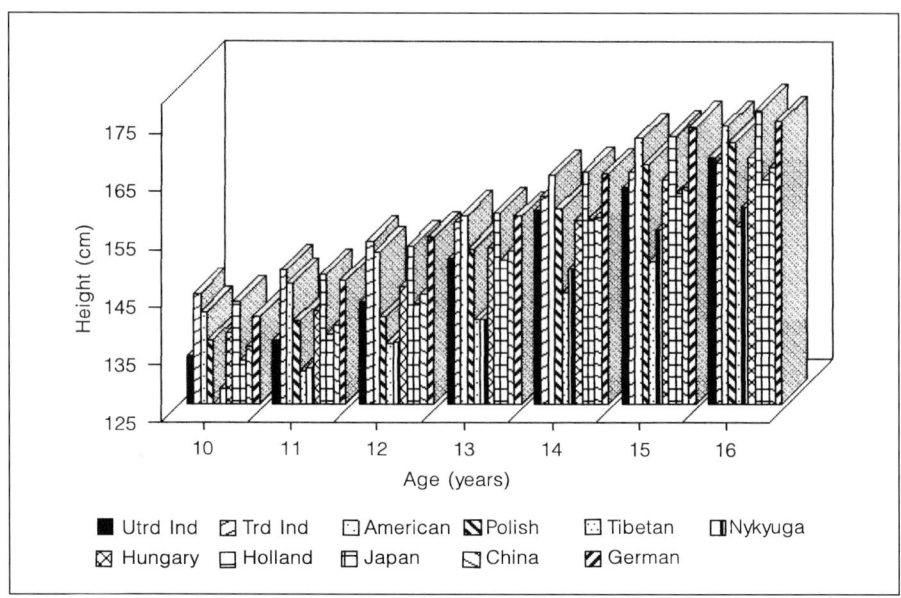

Fig. 2. Comparison of height of Indian children with their international counterparts. Utrd = Untrained; Trd = trained; Ind = Indian.

circulation, muscle blood flow, muscle capillary density, cardiac output, arteriovenous difference and plasma volume [30–33]. Many young children start athletic training and intensive exercise at a young age [34]. Swimming and gymnastic training, for example, often starts as early as 5 or 6 years of age. Although some studies have demonstrated an improvement in aerobic capacity in young children [35–38] other studies of prepubescent children have shown little or no improvement as a result of exercise [39–41].

It is particularly difficult to isolate the effect of exercise on cardiorespiratory factors from the influence of growth, maturation, activity and heredity. However, there is general agreement in the literature that 8- to 13-year-old children are trainable. Pate and Blair [42] reported that improvement in aerobic capacity can occur in prepubescent children provided the training is vigorous and prolonged. Mirwald et al. [43] in a longitudinal study of active and inactive boys aged 7–17 years concluded that activity during preadolescence had no significant effect on aerobic capacity and that puberty was the critical period for increasing maximum aerobic power. Studies of older children suggest that exercise and training which is demanding in intensity, frequency and duration does lead to substantial improvements in cardiorespiratory performance [5, 44–46]. Exercise in adolescents from 14 to 18 years of age produces aerobic

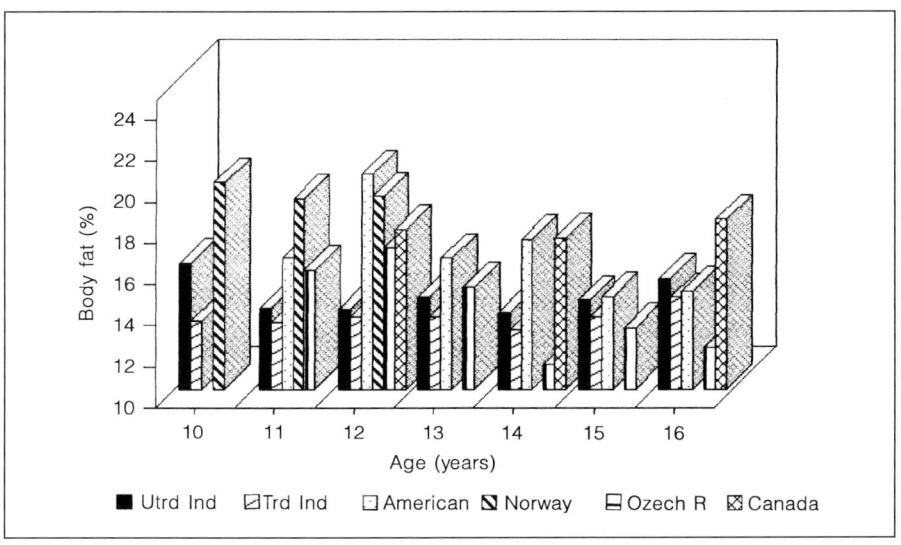

Fig. 3. Comparison of body fat of Indian children with their international counterparts. Utrd = Untrained; Trd = trained; Ind = Indian.

improvements similar to those found in adults. The degree of improvement is dependent upon the level and type of exercise undertaken and the initial fitness of the children [47]. In the present study, the rate of increment of VO_{2max} of trained children was the same as for untrained children. The failure to see a difference may be due to the fact that all are basically active.

Absolute values for maximum O_2 consumption increase as a consequence of increased size [48–50]. Early maturing boys who are bigger in size have greater VO_{2max} mainly as a result of an increase in lean body weight [47]. Maximum aerobic capacity of the trained children are comparable to international counterparts from 13 to 16 years of age (fig. 4) but 10- to 12-year-old children have lower aerobic values compared to Norwegian and Canadian counterparts [43].

Ventilation

There was a nonlinear increase in ventilation of 6.2 and 8.9 liters/min/year in untrained and trained children, respectively. The rate of increase in trained children can be ascribed to better respiratory musculature and lung size [51, 52]. Comparisons with international counterparts revealed that Indian children have lower values for V_{Emax} compared to Canadian children [53], however values are comparable to Japanese children [8] (fig. 5).

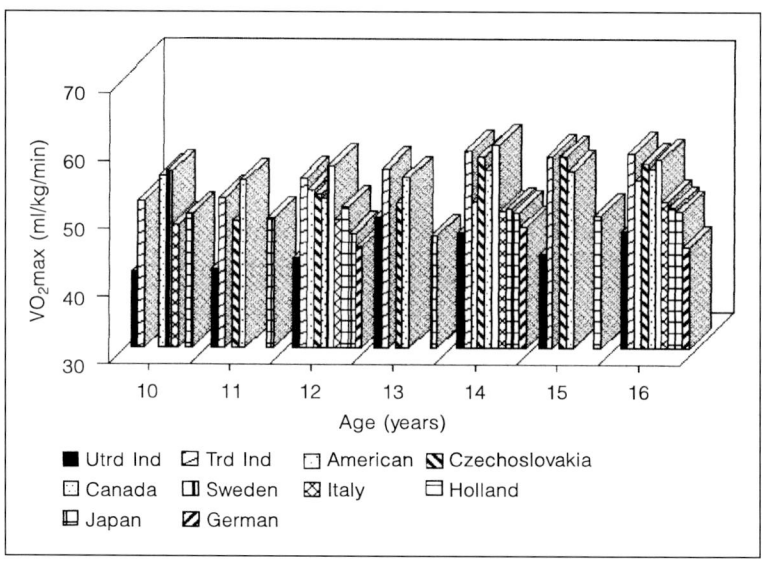

Fig. 4. Comparison of maximum aerobic capacity of Indian children with international counterparts. Utrd = Untrained; Trd = trained; Ind = Indian.

Maximum Heart Rate

Rowland [54] reported that submaximal heart rate falls with increasing age but maximal heart rate remains stable throughout the pediatric years. The untrained children in the present study showed a decreasing trend across the age groups whereas the trained children remained unchanged. Maximum heart rate values are similar to those of Japanese [8], Canadian [53] and Dutch [7]. However, Swedish 12- to 13-year-old children displayed maximum values of 5–10 bpm higher than both groups in the present study. At 15–16 years of age similar values were seen in trained children [1]. Cumming et al. [55] have also reported higher mean heart rates in American children.

O_2 Pulse

Oxygen pulse increases with age in boys because VO_2 increases whilst at the same time, heart rate either remains the same or decreases. Trained individuals have better oxygen pulse values since growth combined with training further improves arteriovenous oxygen content as well as stroke volume, whilst mean value for O_2 pulse is similar in the trained group compared to Dutch children of 12–13 years. However, in the higher age groups the O_2 pulse is lower in Indian children indicating that the rate of development after puberty is not consistent with changes seen in children from developed countries.

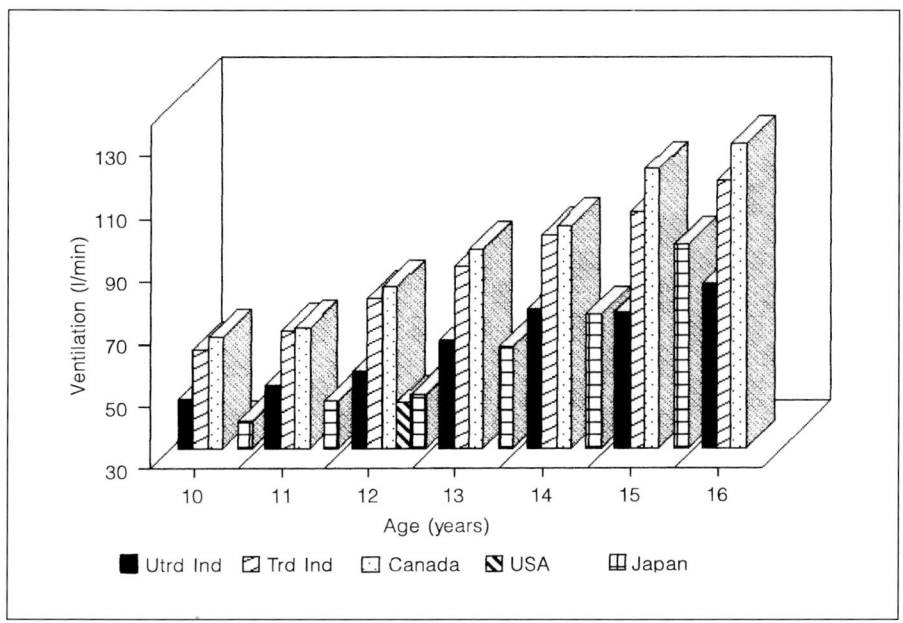

Fig. 5. Comparison of ventilation of Indian children with their international counterparts. Utrd = Untrained; Trd = trained; Ind = Indian.

Similarly, Indian adult sportspersons of various disciplines have lower values than reported for trained German athletes [56].

Anaerobic Capacity

Whilst the O_2 debt is not widely accepted as an indicator of anaerobic capacity, due to its widespread acceptance for many years, it is used in the present study for comparative reasons. Anaerobic capacity is less in children compared to the normal adult population and trained children have a lower O_2 debt as compared to more junior Indian sportspersons [57].

The lower anaerobic capacity of children can be partly explained by their lower level of acidosis at maximum exercise [58]. Sargeant and Dolan [59] suggested that the difference between children and adults depends on the ratio of muscle length to cross-sectional area. The significant difference between groups at 15 and 16 years of age may be due to training enhancing lactate production after peak height velocity. Increases in anaerobic capacity may be due to the effect of dimensional changes in the muscle, the density of the myofibrils, development of neuromuscular transmission and changes in the contractile speed of muscles with growth and training. Each of these factors may contribute to the increase in children's power output and anaerobic component with progressing age.

Summary and Conclusions

Indian children are less developed in physical and physiological components compared to children from various developed countries. This is also true of Indian children selected for high level performance. This may be due to lower socioeconomic status, poor nutritional habits and genetic reasons. Whilst training enhances the development of aerobic and anaerobic capacity, age-specific training programs need to be developed to maximize the gain during the growth and development of children.

References

1   Åstrand PO, Rodahl K: Textbook of Work Physiology. New York, McGraw-Hill, 1986.
2   Sharon AC, William FR, Boileau RA: Metabolic and cardiovascular responses of children during prolonged physical activity. Res Q 1984;55:1–7.
3   Shephard RJ: Fitness of nation, lessons from the Canada fitness survey. Med Sports Sci 1986;22: 186.
4   Máček M, Vávra J: The adjustment of oxygen uptake at the onset of exercise, a comparison between pre-pubertal boys and young adults. Int J Sports Med 1980;1:70–72.
5   Cunnningham DA, Eynon RB: The working capacity of young competitive swimmers 10–16 years of age. Med Sci Sports Exerc 1973;5:227–231.
6   Bonen A, Heywood VH, Cureton KJ, Bioleau RA, Massey BH: Prediction of maximal oxygen uptake in boys, ages 7–15 years. Med Sci Sports 1979;11:24–29.
7   Kemper HCG: Growth, health and fitness of teenagers, longitudinal research in international perspective. Med Sport 1985;20:202.
8   Kobayashi K, Kitamure K, Miura M, Sodeyama H, Murase Y, Miyashita M, Matsui H: Aerobic power as related to body growth and training in Japanese boys: A longitudinal study. J Appl Phys 1978;44:666–672.
9   Matusi H, Miyashita M, Miura M, Amano K, Mizutani S, Hoshikawa T, Toyoshima S, Kamei S: Aerobic work capacity of Japanese adolescents. J Sports Med Phys Fitness 1971;11:28–35.
10 Tanka H, Shindo M: Running velocity at blood lactate threshold of boys aged 6–15 years compared with untrained and trained young males. Int J Sports Med 1985;6:90–94.
11 Pařízková J: Body Fat and Physical Fitness. The Hague, Nijhoff, 1977, p 262.
12 Anderson LB: Changes in physical activity are reflected in changes in fitness during late adolescence: A two year follow up study. J Sports Med Phys Fitness 1994;34:390–397.
13 Khanna GL: Aerobic, Anaerobic Capacities and Cardiopulmonary Responses to Ergometry in Children Ranging in Age from 8 to 18 Years; PhD thesis Punjabi University, Patiala, 1987.
14 Verma SK: Work Capacity and Physiological Responses to Exercise with Special Reference to Age Changes; PhD thesis Punjabi University, Patiala, 1988.
15 Fry EI, Chang KSF, Lee MMC, Ng CK: The amount and distribution of subcutaneous fat tissue in Southern Chinese children from Hong Kong. Am J Phys Anthropol 1965;23:69–80.
16 Malina RM, Bielieu T: Growth and maturation of boys active in sports: Longitudinal observation from the Worclaw growth study. Pediatr Exerc Sci 1992;4:66–77.

17 Pařízková J, Roth Z: The assessment of depot fat in children from skinfold thickness measurements. Hum Biol 1972;44:613–620.
18 Siri WE: Body Composition from Fluid Space and Density Analysis of Methods, in Technique for Measuring Body Composition. Washington, Nat Acad Sci Nat Res Council, 1961.
19 Fox EL, Robinson S, Weigman D: Metabolic energy sources during continuous and interval running. J Appl Phys 1969;27:174–178.
20 Khanna GL, Saha M: Physique and physiological characteristics of Indian National Junior and Senior swimmers with reference to age. NIS Sci J 1992;15:87–95.
21 Singh N: Work Capacity and Cardiorespiratory Adjustments to Exercise in Boys with Special Reference to Age Changes; PhD thesis Punjabi University, Patiala, 1994.
22 ICMR: Growth and Physical Development of Indian Infants and Children. Tech Rep Ser. New Delhi, Pb Ind Coun Med Res, 1984, No 18.
23 Johnson TR, Moore WM, Jeffries JE: Children Are Different: Developmental Physiology, ed 2. Columbus, Ross Laboratories, 1978.
24 Wutscherk H: Grundlagen der Sportsanthropometrie: Messtechnik and Methoden, Leipzig, 1981.
25 Eiben OG: Die körperliche Entwicklung des Kindes; in Willimczik T (ed): Die motorische Entwicklung im Kindes- und Jugendalter. Schorndorf, Hofmann, 1978, pp 187–218.
26 Van Venrooij L, Ijsselmuiden ME: Mixed longitudinal data on height, weight, limb circumference and skinfold measurements of Dutch children. Hum Biol 1978;50:369.
27 Rode A, Shephard RJ: Growth, development and fitness of Canadian Eskimos. Med Sci Sports Exerc 1973;5:161–169.
28 Avlontiou E: Somatic variables for pre-adolescent swimmers. J Sports Med Phys Fitness 1994;34:185–191.
29 Sodhi KS: A Study of Physical Growth and Physical Performance of Punjabi Males Ranging in Age from 8–12 Years with Reference to Their Socioeconomic Status; MD thesis Punjabi University, Patiala, 1993.
30 Chumlea WC, Siervogel RM, Roche AF, Webb P, Rogers E: Increments across age in body composition for children 10–18 years of age. Hum Biol 1983;55:845–852.
31 Lewis DA, Kama E, Hodgson JL: Physiological differences between genders: Implicatioins for sports conditioning. Sports Med 1986;3:357.
32 Vaccaro P, Mahon A: Cardiorespiratory responses to endurance training in children. Sports Med 1987;4:352–363.
33 Armstrong N, Welsoman JR: Assessment and interpretation of aerobic fitness in children and adolescents. Exerc Sport Sci Rev 1994;22:435–476.
34 Sady SP: Cardiorespiratory exercise in children; in Katch F, Freedson P (eds): Clinics in Sports Medicine. Philadelphia, Sauders, 1986, p 493.
35 Brown CH, Harrower JR, Deeter MF: The effects of cross country running on pre-adolescent girls. Med Sci Sports Exerc 1972;4:1–5.
36 Eriksson BO, Koch G: Effect of physical training on haemodynamic response during sub-maximal exercise in 11–13 year old boys. Acta Physiol Scand 1973;87:27–39.
37 Lussier L, Buskirk ER: Effect of endurance training programme on assessment of work capacity in pre-pubertal children. Ann NY Acad Sci 1977;301:734.
38 Yoshizawa S, Ishizaki T, Honda H: Aerobic power and endurance running in young children; in Rutenfranz J, et al (eds): Children and Exercise. Champaign, Human Kinetics, 1986, vol 12, p 77.
39 Stewart K, Gutin B: Effects of physical training on cardiorespiratory fitness in children. Res Q 1976;47:110–120.
40 Mckeag DB: Longitudinal cardiorespiratory performance testing in young swimmers; in Brown EW, Branta CF (eds): Competitive Sport for Children and Youth. Champaign, Human Kinetics, 1988, p 259.
41 Bar-Or O: Pediatric Sports Medicine for the Practitioner. New York, Springer, 1983, p 30.
42 Pate RR, Blair SN: Exercise and the prevention of atherosclerosis: Pediatric implications; in Strong WB (ed): Atherosclerosis: Its Pediatric Aspects. New York, Grune & Stralton, 1978.
43 Mirwald RL, Bailey DA, Cameron N, Rasmussen RL: Longitudinal comparison of aerobic power in active and inactive boys aged 7 to 17 years. Ann Hum Biol 1981;8:405–414.

44 Koch G: Lung dimensions, ventilatory capacity and muscle blood flow in 12–16 year old boys with high physical activity; in Ber K, Eriksson BO (eds): Children and Exercise. Baltimore, University Park Press, 1980, vol 9, p 99.
45 Placheta Z: Youth and Physical Activity, Brno, JE Purkyně University, 1980.
46 Vaccaro P, Clarke DH, Morries AF: Physiological characteristics of young well trained swimmers. Eur J Appl Physiol 1980;44:61.
47 Bale P: The functional performance of children in relation to growth, maturation and exercise. Sports Med 1992;3:151–159.
48 Åstrand PO: The child in sport and physical activity; in Albinson JG, Andrew GM (eds): Child in Sport and Physical Activity. International Series on Sports Science. Baltimore, University Park Press, 1977, vol 3, pp 19–33.
49 Armstrong N, Davies B: The metabolic and physiological responses of children to exercise and training. Phys Educ Rev 1984;7:90–94.
50 Borms J: The child and exercise: An overview. J Sports Sci 1986;4:3–20.
51 Robinson EP, Kjeldgaard JM: Improvement in ventilatory muscle function with running. J Appl Physiol 1982;52:1400–1406.
52 Lakhera SC, Kaiu TC, Bandopadhay P: Changes in lung function during adolescence in athletes and non-athletes. J Sports Med Phys Fitness 1994;34:258–262.
53 Massicotte DR, Gauthier R, Markon P: Prediction of VO_2max from running performance in children aged 10–17 years. J Sports Med Phys Fitness 1985;25:10–17.
54 Rowland TW: Exercise and Children's Health. Champaign, Human Kinetics, 1990, pp 80–84.
55 Cumming GR, Everatt D, Hastonan L: Bruce treadmill test in children: Normal values in a clinic population. Am J Cardiol 1978;41:69–75.
56 Hollmann W, Barg W, Weyer G, Heck H: Age influence on the spiroergometric measurements in submaximal region (in German). Med Welt 1970;28:1280–1288.
57 Khanna GL, Dey SK, Batra M, Saha M: Applied physiology of sports: Indian National sportspersons. Bangalore, Pb Sports Authority of India, 1991, pp 1–54.
58 Inbar O, Bar-Or O: Anaerobic characteristics in male children and adolescents. Med Sci Sports Exerc 1984;18:264–267.
59 Sargeant AJ, Dolan P: Optimal velocity of muscle contraction for short-term (anaerobic) power output in children and adults; in Rutenfranz J (ed): Children and Exercise. Champaign, Human Kinetics, 1986, vol 12, pp 39–42.

Dr G.L. Khanna, Scientific Officer, Head Department of Exercise Physiology,
Faculty of Sports Sciences, Sports Authority of India, Netaji Subhas Southern Centre,
Bangalore – 560 056 (India)

Treatment and Prevention of Obesity by Exercise in Czech Children

Jana Pařízková

Laboratory of Health Promotion, 1st Medical Faculty, Charles University, Prague, Czech Republic

Introduction

The increasing prevalence of obesity in children and adolescents has been mainly explained by a decreased level of physical activity and energy output [1–5]. Lower levels of physical activity also have a significant impact on the level of functional capacity, especially of the cardiorespiratory system, which is further related to the actual and future health risks [4, 6–8]. Whilst fewer preschool-aged children are obese compared to school age and adolescents, the negative impact of excess fatness is already apparent in young children and varies according to different items of physical fitness and motor performance [4].

The reduction of food intake below recommended daily allowances (RDAs) is not indicated as a prevention and treatment of obesity in children as this may slow down the growth in height [2, 3]. The correction of any energy imbalance by increasing the energy output by suitable exercise is therefore recommended as the most effective method of treatment during the growing years [3].

Subjects and Methods

Several groups of children and youths from 8 to 14 years of age were followed up during various phases of obesity, before and after treatment in the Outpatient Department for Obese Children. The following morphologic and functional variables were estimated: body mass index (BMI, standards for the Czech population were used) [9], body composition,

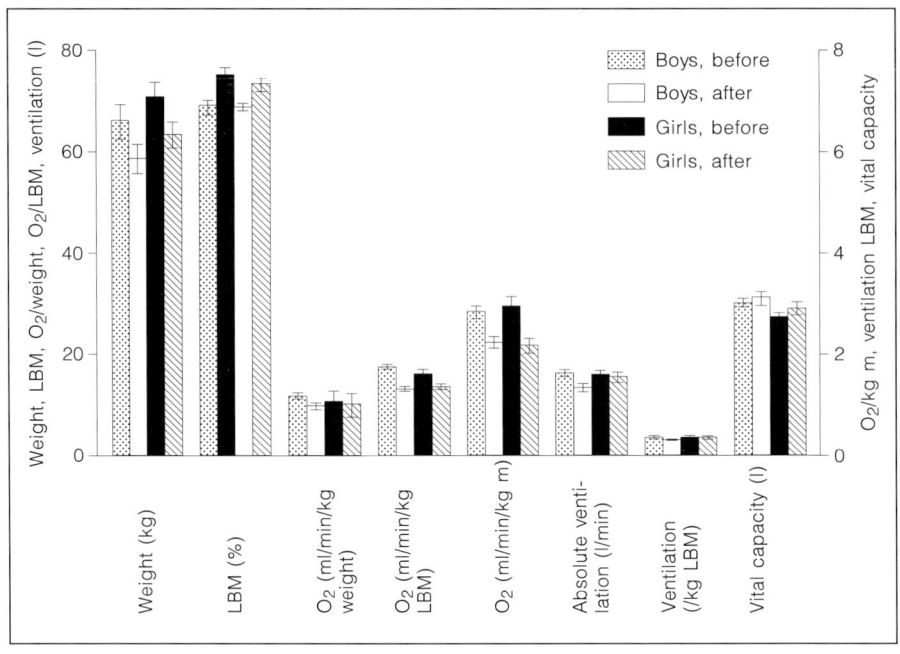

Fig. 1. Changes of body weight, percentage of LBM, absolute and relative values of the oxygen uptake during standard workload on a veloergometer in obese boys (n = 18) and girls (n = 15) before and after the reduction of weight and depot fat in a special summer training camp (7 weeks; mean values ± SE).

that is the absolute and relative amounts of lean body mass (LBM) and depot fat using densitometry (with simultaneous measurements of the air in the lungs and respiratory passages), aerobic power assessed during a maximal workload on a treadmill (max O_2), and performance during the standard workload (estimated as one third of the max O_2), on a veloergometer. Serum cholesterol was also assessed [2].

The results were compared before and after treatment in a summer camp lasting 50 days. Measurements were undertaken either during 1 year, or repeatedly across a 2- to 4-year period during which children successively attended the abovementioned summer camps. The treatment consisted of (1) a monitored diet of approximately 4,000 kJ, with an adequate composition (proteins, minerals and vitamins according to RDAs), reduced fat, an increased amount of vegetables and fruit, and 1.5 liters of unsweetened beverages per day; (2) an exercise program conducted each day and modified according to the individual capabilities of the child; for heavier individuals, exercise was commenced in the sitting position, and this was followed later by weight-bearing exercises; a wide range of attractive sports activities were introduced and supervised by experienced staff, and (3) behavioral intervention.

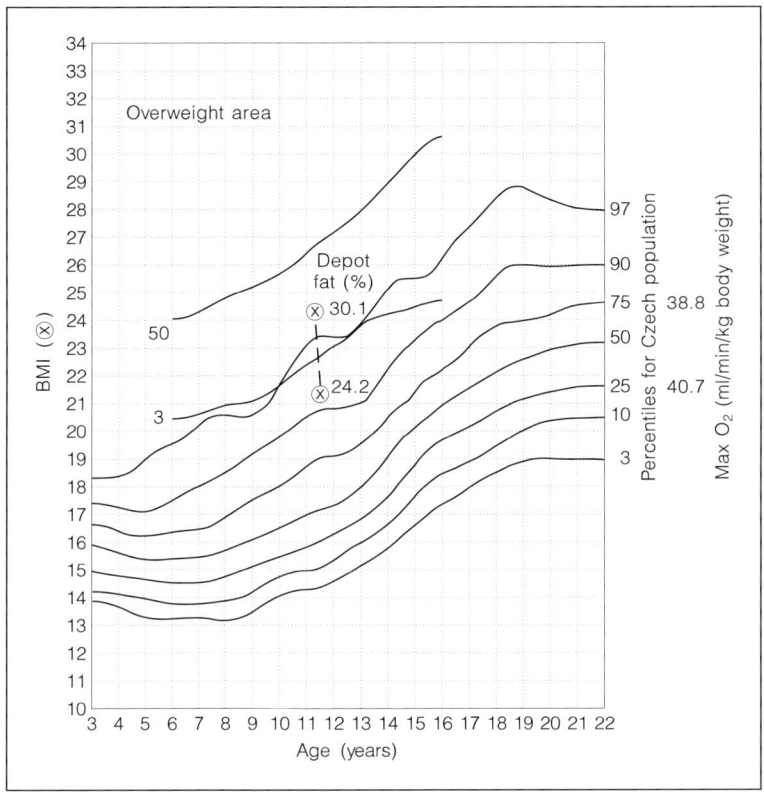

Fig. 2. Changes of BMI, percentage of depot fat (hydrodensitometry) and aerobic power in a group of 7 obese boys before and after reduction of weight and of depot fat in a special summer training camp. A lowering of BMI along with the reduction of the percentage of depot fat and simultaneous significant increase of the aerobic power (lower value before reduction of BMI and fat, higher value after reduction, indicating the increase of the aerobic power after reduction treatment in summer camp) is shown. Lines in overweight area of the grid, 50th and 3rd percentiles for the obese population, as measured by Bláha [9].

Results

Comparisons of functional capacity between obese subjects and normal weight children of the same age showed consistently lower levels of performance in the obese. Dynamic weight-bearing activities of an aerobic nature showed the most pronounced differences. The obese were not disadvantaged in muscular strength [2].

Body weight, fat mass (kg) and BMI significantly decreased in the first group of obese boys and girls following treatment in the camp whilst relative

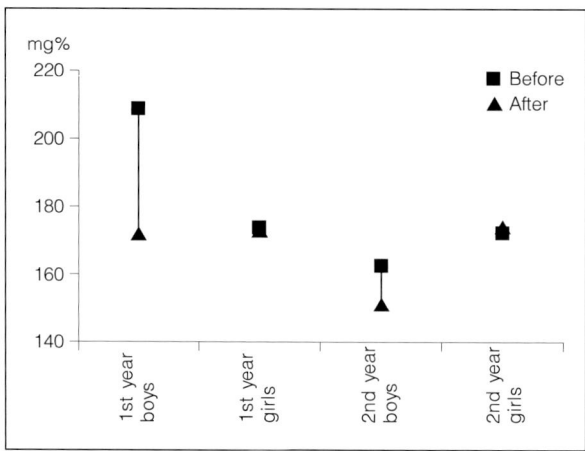

Fig. 3. Changes of blood cholesterol in obese boys and girls before and after the reduction of body weight and of depot fat in a special summer training camp in 2 consecutive years.

LBM (%) increased. The standard physical workload on a bicycle ergometer was performed more economically after weight and fat reduction. That is, oxygen uptake related to total and lean body mass, and to kilogram meters of performance decreased as did ventilation in absolute values and per kilogram of LBM. Vital capacity increased. All changes were statistically significant (fig. 1).

Maximal oxygen uptake per kilogram body weight increased significantly following the program (fig. 2). Concomitant with the increase in aerobic power was a significant decline in the level of total serum cholesterol. However, the changes were more apparent in boys whose initial levels were higher than in girls (fig. 3).

The same groups of children were also followed before and after a similar summer camp treatment the following year. The level of cholesterol did not increase in these children during the school year in spite of an increase in BMI and body fat. A further significant decline of total serum cholesterol was observed after the second summer camp in boys.

In some children, the results of the treatment were not permanent. An increase in height during the school year and corresponding increases in BMI and body fat meant that these children were under permanent supervision in the Outpatient Department for Obese Children. A small group of boys (n = 8) was followed during 4 consecutive years during which they attended four summer treatment camps. In this group there were yearly fluctuations in

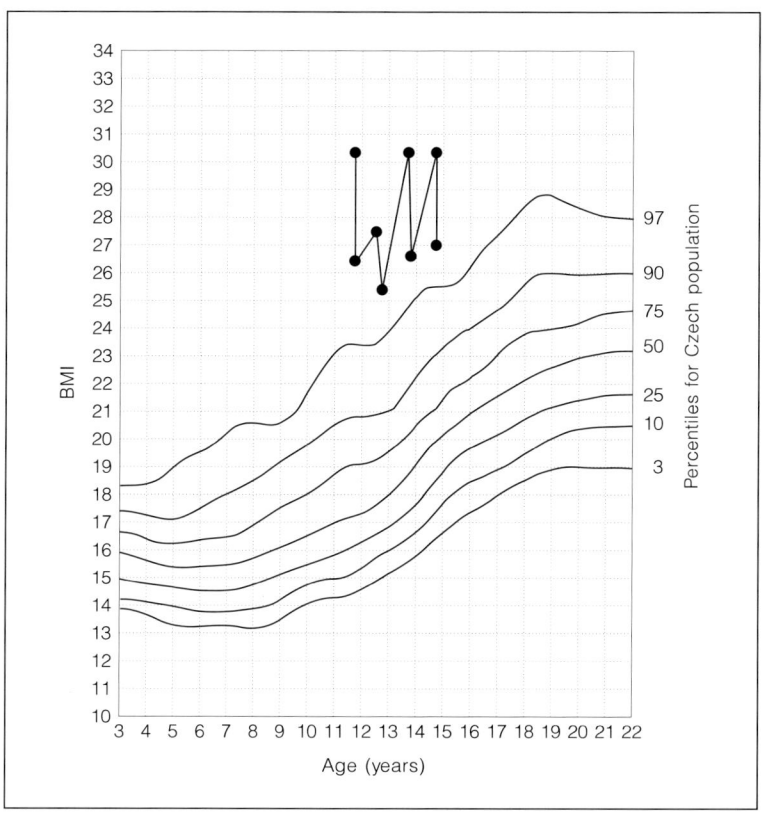

Fig. 4. Longitudinal study of BMI in a group of obese boys (n = 8) during the reduction treatment in 4 consecutive summer training camps (monitored diet approximately 4,000 kJ/day + exercise); curve (●) in the upper part of the grid.

weight, fat and BMI (fig. 4) which did not normalize but moved closer to standard values after repeated treatment. Simultaneous controls of body composition using densitometry showed a significant increase of LBM which did not decrease after summer camp treatment when the boys were younger (fig. 5). A slight decrease in LBM was apparent during the last 2 years after treatment. LBM was significantly greater in obese than normal weight boys of the same age and height. The percent body fat of participants always decreased significantly following the reduction treatment, but increased again during the school year. However, the long-term trend of this 4-year treatment program was positive, that is the absolute and relative amount of fat decreased significantly.

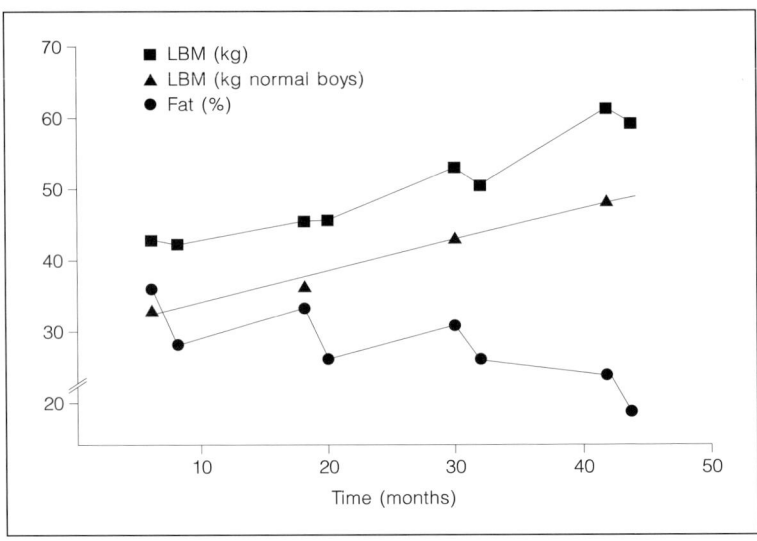

Fig. 5. Longitudinal study of the changes of body composition (kg LBM, percentage of depot fat by hydrodensitometry) in a group of obese boys during the reduction treatment in 4 consecutive summer training camps.

As for other measurements, functional testing on a bicycle ergometer showed a significant decline in oxygen uptake, that is lower energy output during the same or increasing work performance (kg m) plus an improved mechanical efficiency and economy of work. Heart rate levels during this standard workload of lower intensity remained the same during the 4-year period (fig. 6).

A subject who initially presented with morbid obesity had outstanding success reducing BMI and depot fat due to an excellent maintenance of exercise and diet, even during the school year (fig. 7).

Discussion

Increased levels of physical activity and regular exercise reduce body fat which is apparent in preschool-aged children [10, 11]. Exercise is therefore recommended not only for the prevention of obesity, but also as the most efficient tool for the reduction of BMI and percentage of depot fat, and for the improvement of physical fitness and work performance [2]. A range of studies have shown that early intervention can have a significant effect [3, 4, 12, 13, 17].

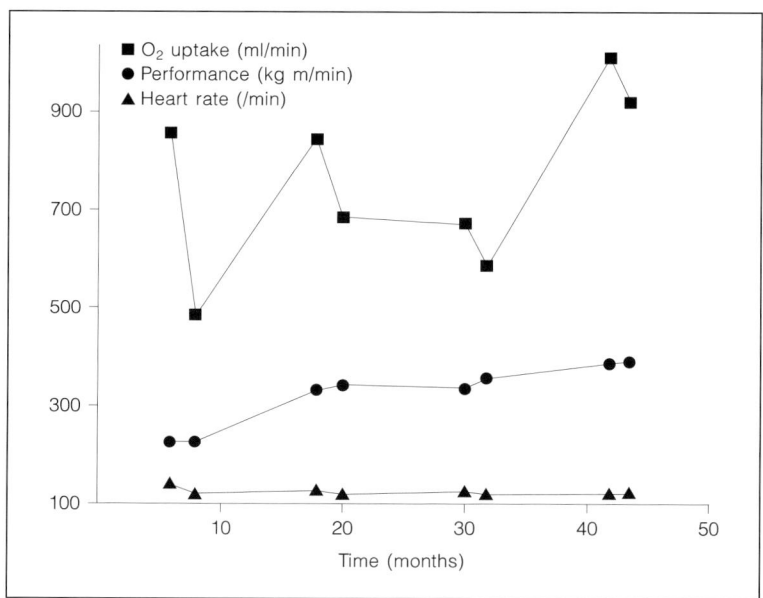

Fig. 6. Longitudinal study of the oxygen uptake, heart rate and work performance during a standard workload in a group of obese boys during the reduction treatment in 4 consecutive summer training camps.

Measurements in the current study revealed the same absolute values of aerobic power characterized by max O_2 ($l \cdot min^{-1}$) in obese and nonobese children. A similar result was shown by Maffeis et al. [14]. However, when aerobic power was related to body weight, the values in the obese were significantly lower indicating a lower level of cardiorespiratory efficiency manifested especially during weight-bearing activities such as longer runs. The reduction of body weight and fatness after treatment in summer camps improved the level of fitness and physical performance. Following reduction, values of max O_2 ($ml \cdot kg^{-1} \cdot min^{-1}$) in obese boys increased significantly and physical working capacity improved with longer running times achieved at higher speeds. Improvement was also evident in a variety of sporting activities at the end of the summer camps. Similar long-term studies assessing body composition, aerobic power, physical performance and serum lipids before and after repeated weight and fat reduction periods in growing children are uncommon [8]. Similar to results with adults, exercise significantly improved serum cholesterol levels. This was particularly apparent in boys whose cholesterol levels were elevated [7].

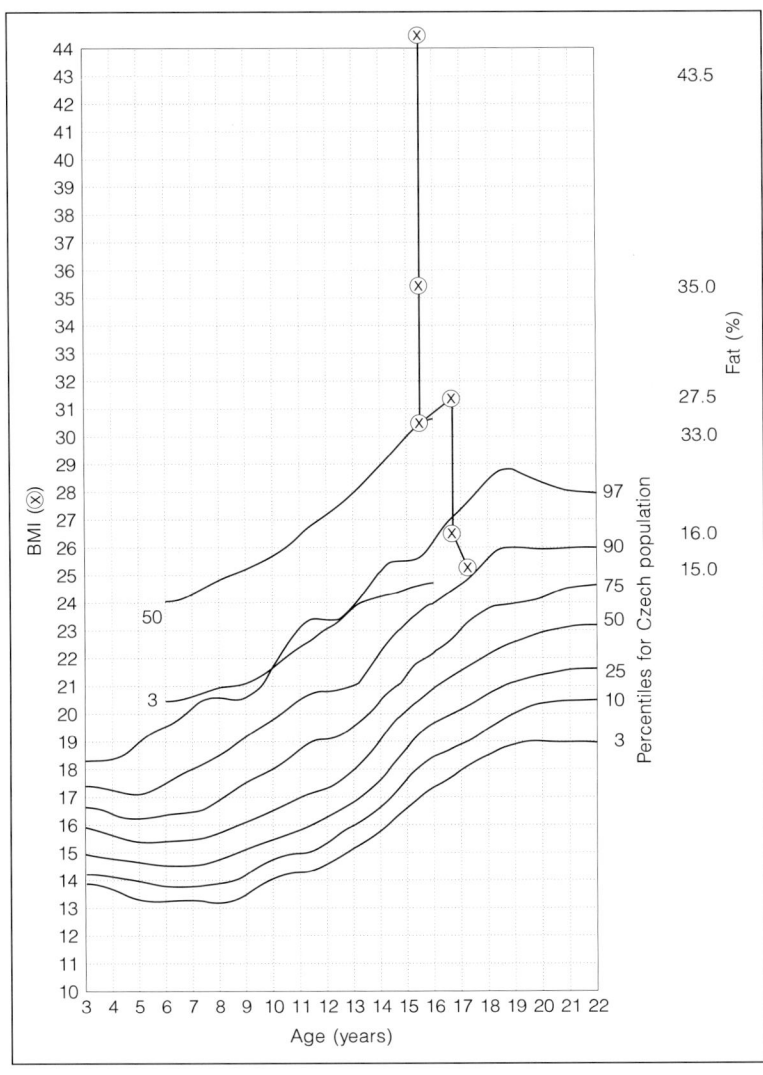

Fig. 7. Changes of BMI and the percentage of depot fat in an obese boy during 2 years of reduction treatment in two summer training camps and in the Outpatient Department of the Children's Clinic.

Weight cycling characteristics were manifested during growth in a number of children. A sustained regime of exercise along with a monitored diet are the necessary prerequisites for the preservation of the positive results of the summer camps. Adherence to a monitored diet that involves other members of the family who are often not obese, along with sufficient exercise every (or most) day(s) during the school year is extremely difficult. There were only a small number of individuals who were able to maintain body weight and fat reduction at home. This success was limited to older subjects.

Repeated measurements of subjects across a 4-year period revealed that the treatment in summer camps did not reduce LBM in younger subjects before puberty (fig. 5) which is often a common characteristic [3, 15]. Clearly, the treatment of obesity must be commenced as early as possible [4, 11, 12, 16, 17]. An appropriate lifestyle with an adequate diet and physical activity regime is, however, the best way to prevent the development of obesity in early childhood.

Summary and Conclusions

Exercise therapy with a monitored diet in special summer camps lasting several weeks appears to be a sound procedure for reduction of weight and fatness in children and youth as simultaneously the level of physical fitness was improved. Improvement was also established in aerobic power (max O_2), economy of work, performance in various sport disciplines (running, swimming, climbing, participation in various games) and reduction of serum cholesterol.

Measurements of body composition confirmed that it is imperative that such treatment is commenced as early as possible but definitely prior to puberty when LBM does not decrease during such a treatment regime. In contrast to the methodology described in this study, outpatient treatment is usually not as effective even when the same principles are employed. Best results were obtained when children were able to attend summer camps during consecutive years. This helped in the habituation of diet, exercise and behaviors.

A further advantage of the abovementioned treatment regime was the manner in which children embraced the activity program. Children enjoyed the program and were relatively uninhibited in the camp environment compared with the usual conditions throughout the school year. A permanent change in behavior and related positive results during the balance of the school year very much depends on the active support and encouragement of the child's family. Nevertheless, marked improvements are possible for highly motivated young subjects even under the usual conditions of life, provided that a real effort is made to complete sufficient exercise and a suitable diet is adhered to.

References

1 Durnin JVGA, Lonergan ME, Good J, Ewan A: A cross-sectional nutritional and anthropometric study with an interval of 7 years on 611 young adolescent schoolchildren. Br J Nutr 1974;32: 169–179.
2 Pařízková J: Body Fat and Physical Fitness. Body Composition and Lipid Metabolism in Different Regimes of Physical Activity. The Hague, Nijhoff, 1977.
3 Pařízková J: Obesity and its treatment by diet and exercise; in Simopoulos A (ed): Nutrition and Fitness in Health and Diseases. World Rev Nutr Diet. Basel, Karger, 1993, vol 72, pp 78–91.
4 Pařízková J: Nutrition, Physical Activity, and Health in Early Life. Boca Raton, CRC Press, 1996.
5 Donnelly JE, Jacobsen DJ, Whatley JE, Hill JO, Swift LL, Cherrington A, Polk B, Tran ZV, Reed G: Nutrition and physical activity program to attenuate and promote physical and metabolic fitness in elementary school children. Obes Res 1996;4:229–243.
6 Schlicker SA, Borra ST, Regan C: The weight and fitness status of United States children. Nutr Rev 1994;52:11–17.
7 Berg A, Halle M, Bauer S, Korsten-Reck V, Keul J: Körperliche Aktivität und Essverhalten: Strategien zur Verbesserung des Serumlipidprofils bei Kindern und Jugendlichen. Wien Med Wochenschr 1994;144:138–144.
8 Hills AP, Wahlqvist ML: Exercise and Obesity. London, Smith-Gordon, 1994.
9 Bláha P: W/H^2 Body Mass Index of the Current Czechoslovak Population between the Ages of 3 to 70. Prague, Institute of Sports Medicine, 1991.
10 Pařízková J, Macková E, Kábele J, Macková J, Škopková M: Body composition, food intake, cardiorespiratory fitness, blood lipids and psychological development in highly active and inactive preschool children. Hum Biol 1986;58:261.
11 Davies PSW, Gregory J, Whitte A: Physical activity and body fatness in preschool children. Int J Obes 1995;19:6.
12 Davies PSW, Christoffel KK: Obesity in preschool and school-age children. Treatment early and often may be best. Arch Pediatr Adolesc Med 1994;148:125.
13 Harsha DW: The benefits of physical activity in childhood. Am J Med Sci 1995;310(suppl 1): S109–S113.
14 Maffeis C, Schena F, Zafanello M, Zoccante L, Schutz Y, Pinelli L: Maximal aerobic power during running and cycling in obese and non-obese children. Acta Paediatr 1994;83:113–116.
15 Pařízková J, Hainer V: Exercise in growing and adult obese individuals; in Torg JS, Welsh RP, Shephard RJ(eds): Current Therapy in Sports Medicine. Toronto, Decker, 1990, p 22.
16 Klish WJ: Childhood obesity: Pathophysiology and treatment. Acta Paediatr Jpn 1995;37:1–6.
17 Pařízková J: Interaction between physical activity and nutrition early in life and their impact on later development. Nutr Res Rev 1998;11:1–21.

Assoc. Prof. Jana Pařízková, MD, PhD, DSc, Laboratory of Health Promotion,
3rd Clinic of Internal Medicine, 1st Medical School, Charles University,
U Nemocnice 2, CZ–12806 Prague 2 (Czech Republic)
Fax + +420-2 295870 or home 299496
E-Mail parizek@mbox.cesnet.cz

Methodological Considerations in the Assessment of Physical Activity and Nutritional Status of Children and Youth

Andrew P. Hills[a], Nuala M. Byrne[a], Jana Pařízková[b]

[a] School of Human Movement Studies, Queensland University of Technology, Brisbane, Australia;
[b] Laboratory of Health Promotion, 3rd Clinic of Internal Medicine, 1st Medical School, Charles University, Prague, Czech Republic

Introduction

The body of knowledge regarding nutrition and physical activity and the effects on health and well-being is well developed but our understanding is still deficient in many areas. The numerous challenges for researchers interested in the assessment of nutritional status, growth, maturation or physical fitness often include methodological concerns. Methodological challenges may occur at all levels in the research process, from the time of instrument choice, through to data collection and analysis. Further, attempts to compare the findings of one study with the literature may be compromised due to peculiarities in the available historical data.

From an international perspective, the conduct of research in different environments, with the associated diversity of resources, plus cultural, climatic and racial uniqueness, can magnify the potential challenges. Whenever possible, common methodological approaches should be pursued to maximize the utility of data.

The aim of this chapter is to address some of the fundamental methodological considerations that have a bearing upon the assessment of nutritional status and physical activity in a range of settings, with specific reference to children and youth. A number of key review documents will be referenced to provide the reader with further content in this important area.

Reliability, Validity and Efficacy

The major considerations in the choice of a method or technique include the reliability, validity and efficacy of the instrument. Reliability (or repeatability, reproducibility) is the extent to which a method produces similar values on two or more occasions [1] and may be expressed in terms of intra- or inter-tester repeatability. Precision and accuracy are often used to reference the ability of a measurement technique to produce a constant or stable value or the ability of a measurement system to achieve the 'right' answer. The reliability of a measurement or method is immaterial if the methodology is not valid. Validity refers to the extent to which the measurement or method is a true indication of the variable being assessed. Further, the generalizability or efficacy of a methodology is critical. A particular measurement protocol may have an acceptable reliability and validity but may not be an appropriate measure for all groups.

Key Issues and Related Questions

The following outline is a compilation of key issues and related questions that may be applied to the measurement of a range of biological parameters [Norgan, unpubl. data, 2]. They may be used as a primer, a guide to some of the numerous questions that one may ask as part of the decision making related to the utilization of a particular methodology.

Rationale for the choice of a particular methodology
What variable is to be measured?
What is the relevance of the measurement?
How important is the measurement?

Issues of precision and accuracy
Who is measuring?
Who is being measured?
What are the expected changes or differences?
Does reference data exist to enable comparisons of data sets?

Choice of equipment
How practical is the technique, equipment or apparatus?
Is the cost prohibitive?
Does the use of the equipment present particular technical difficulties?
How is maintenance and calibration between testing sessions to be managed?

Acceptability of the methodology to subjects
Is the methodology time efficient?
Is it easy to use and nonthreatening to subjects?
How appropriate is the measure? Appropriateness relates to considerations of population differences in age, ethnicity or geographical region [1].

Important Reading

The reader is encouraged to access additional, more comprehensive examples from the literature in both the nutrition [1–11] and physical activity domains [1, 11–20]. These include an extensive measurement overview by Baranowski and Simons-Morton [1] on dietary and physical activity assessment. This paper considers reliability and validity from the perspective of prior assessment, precision, appropriateness, implementation and costs. The paper is the introduction to a complete issue of the *Journal of School Health* [11] devoted to measurement of diet and physical activity. A comprehensive review and evaluation of laboratory and field techniques for physical activity and energy expenditure measurement by Montoye et al. [15] are also a valuable resource. The book highlights examples of future research to improve the validity and precision of methods in these areas. For researchers interested in longitudinal research, the proceedings of a symposium on Problems and Solutions in Longitudinal Research [16] is an important document. Other useful sources include the US Surgeon General's Report on Physical Activity and Health [17], an issue of the journal *Pediatric Exercise Science* devoted to Physical Activity Guidelines for Adolescents [18] and an issue of *Medicine and Science in Sports and Exercise* entitled A Collection of Physical Activity Questionnaires for Health-Related Research [19]. These suggestions are by no means exclusive but do provide an important starting point for extra reading.

Last century, Beneke (1878) is reported to have said that nothing is measured with greater error than the human body. This comment may still be true today in relation to some anthropometric measures and also reflects the assumptions that are made regarding the use and interpretation of particular methodologies. It is critical that researchers do not make rash decisions in respect of choice of methods. No single method is best for all circumstances but it is important to recognize that there are appropriate methods for particular studies [1].

A more complex and/or expensive instrument, whether this be a questionnaire or piece of technology, does not guarantee immunity from assessment problems. For example, a supposedly simple anthropometric measurement protocol may provide as many methodological challenges as a more complex laboratory-based procedure in the assessment of body composition. The range of measurement options available, and acceptable derivatives of the same measurement mean that comparisons between research findings conducted by different groups in a range of physical locations are often difficult.

The methodologies employed in nutritional assessment vary according to the nature of the assessment, that is whether it is community- or group-based as opposed to an individual assessment. There is overlap here with physical activity and physical fitness derivatives. According to the Royal Australasian College of Physicians [21], a comprehensive assessment of nutrition should include the sociocultural role of food, food beliefs, nutrition knowledge and skills, food intake, energy expenditure and the relationship of these factors to performance, morbidity and mortality. At an individual level, assessment should ideally comprise an anthropometric protocol, for example, stature, body mass, girths and skin fold thickness plus a consideration of energy balance through food intake and physical activity measures.

In the childhood years the two primary indicators of growth status, and the most common anthropometric measures are stature (standing height) and body mass (body weight). Accurate measurement of these variables provides a good understanding of maturation and nutritional status and a basis of comparison between individuals of the same chronological age. Individual growth patterns and gender differences based on distance or velocity measures of height and weight are particularly valuable outcomes, but only if measurements have been completed with precision and accuracy. Subsequent comparisons with reference standards may or may not be possible for particular populations. One may need to refer to growth charts produced by the World Health Organisation to gain reference values that have application to a wide range of populations.

In the field of anthropometry, the International Society for the Advancement of Kinanthropometry (ISAK) has made significant advances in recent years in an attempt to bring a more consistent approach to anthropometric measurement technique. This has extended to the provision of various levels of accreditation for anthropometry, graded according to criterion anthropometrists. The developments in this field have been referenced in a recent monograph [22].

Some studies concerning the impact of malnutrition on somatic and fitness development, for example in the countries of the Third World, recommend the comparison of morphological characteristics with functional status. Quite often, smaller marginally malnourished children achieve satisfactory results for physical fitness, which may be the same, or even better than results achieved by bigger peers with superior nutrition in the industrially developed countries. Therefore, local standards and norms for somatic development are recommended as the differences in the 'optimal' or 50th percentile values of height, weight and body mass index can vary in children with very similar and/or corresponding health and fitness development. There have been instances, for example from Africa and New Guinea, where smaller subjects recorded high levels of fitness, but according to all international standards would be characterized as unfit. For these reasons, the evaluation of functional capacity and physical fitness is so important. This issue is another critical goal for researchers everywhere, but especially in the developing countries. Unfortunately, the measurement of physical fitness is often only perceived as important if it relates to sports activities. This notion is totally wrong, all researchers interested in health, nutrition and human development should pay more attention to the aspects mentioned above.

The assessment of the fitness level of an individual, and each of the characteristics most closely related to one's functional capacity (especially such as anthropometry which may be attained under field conditions) have central importance. This is true not only for the comprehensive evaluation of an individual's current developmental level, but perhaps more importantly, has more far-reaching implications for health promotion. These include the potential longer-term benefits for later periods in life. The World Health Organization publication on Prevention in Childhood and Youth of Adult Cardiovascular Diseases: Time for Action [23] stressed the importance of adequate physical activity combined with a desirable diet as one of the preventive measures against adult health problems, and an important goal for a whole-of-life health promotion and the development of positive health. An optimal physical acivity regime alongside an adequate nutrition must be commenced early in life [24, 25]. Consequently, it is essential for measurement tools to be simple and reliable as well as being applicable for use in a wide range of conditions all round the world.

Conclusion

There are many opportunities for additional research to assess and refine existing methodologies. Further, there is an urgent need for new techniques to be devised that are appropriate to the abilities and requirements of particular populations, for example disability groups. Too often, existing instruments are used or modifications are made to such instruments in the hope that they will be applicable to other populations, without due consideration of the implications of this approach. In a similar vein, adult assessment techniques are routinely but inappropriately employed in analyses involving children and youth.

References

1 Baranowski T, Simons-Morton BG: Dietary and physical activity assessment in school-aged children: Measurement issues. J Sch Health 1990;61:195–197.
2 Durnin JVGA: Appropriate technology in body composition: A brief review. Asia Pac J Clin Nutr 1995;4:1–5.
3 Program Evaluation Handbook: Nutrition Education. Atlanta, Centers for Disease Control, 1988, pp 1–206.
4 Simons-Morton BG, Baranowski T: Observation in assessment of children's dietary practices. J Sch Health 1990;61/5:204–207.

5 Lohman TG: Advances in Body Composition Assessment. Champaign, Human Kinetics, 1994.
6 Kral JG, VanItallie TB: Recent Developments in Body Composition Analysis: Methods and Applications. London, Smith-Gordon, 1993.
7 Heyward VH, Stolarczyk LM: Applied Body Composition Assessment. Champaign, Human Kinetics, 1996.
8 Cheung LWY, Richmond JB: Child Health, Nutrition, and Physical Activity. Champaign, Human Kinetics, 1995.
9 Byrne NM, Hills AP: Assessment of eating practices in adolescence. Proc Nutr Soc Aust 1995;19:104.
10 Williamson DA: Assessment of Eating Disorders. Obesity, Anorexia and Bulimia nervosa. New York, Pergamon Press, 1990.
11 Simons-Morton BG, Baranowski T: Dietary and physical activity assessment in school-aged children. J Sch Health 1990;61/5:191–222.
12 Sallis JF: Self-report measures of children's physical activity. J Sch Health 1990;61/5:215–219.
13 Docherty D: Measurement in Pediatric Exercise Science. Champaign, Human Kinetics, 1996.
14 Blimkie CJR, Bar-Or O: New Horizons in Pediatric Exercise Science. Champaign, Human Kinetics, 1995.
15 Montoye HJ, Kemper HCG, Saris WHM, Washburn RA: Measuring Physical Activity and Energy Expenditure. Champaign, Human Kinetics, 1996.
16 Kemper HCG, van Mechelen W, Mellenbergh GJ: Problems and solutions in longitudinal research. Int J Sports Med 1997;18(suppl 3):S139–S254.
17 Physical Activity and Health: A report of the Surgeon General US Department of Health and Human Services, Centers for Disease Control, 1996.
18 Sallis JF: Physical activity guidelines for adolescents. Pediatr Exerc Sci 1994;6:299–471.
19 Kriska AM, Caspersen CJ: A collection of physical activity questionnaires for health-related research. Med Sci Sports Exerc 1997;29(suppl 6):S1–S205.
20 Sallis JF, Patrick K: Physical activity guidelines for adolescents: Consensus statement. Pediatr Exerc Sci 1994;6:302–314.
21 Royal Australasian College of Physicians: Responsibility for Nutrition Diagnosis. London, Smith-Gordon, 1989.
22 Norton K, Olds T: Anthropometrica. Sydney, University of New South Wales Press, 1996.
23 World Health Oganization: Prevention in childhood and youth of adult cardiovascular diseases. Technical Report of WHO Expert Committee. Tech Rep Ser. Geneva, WHO, 1990, No 792.
24 Pařízková J: How much energy is consumed and spent for optimal growth and development? Nutrition 1996;12:820–821.
25 Pařízková J: Interaction between physical activity and nutrition early in life and their impact on later development. Nutr Res Rev 1998;11:1–21.

Associate Professor A.P. Hills, School of Human Movement Studies,
Queensland University of Technology, Victoria Park Road,
Brisbane, Kelvin Grove, QLD 4059 (Australia)

Conclusions and Perspectives

This monograph presents a diversity of information relating to nutrition and physical fitness. As the title suggests, the volume is truly representative of the current status of a number of groups of children and youth living in a wide range of physical environments. It is significant that the chapters provide an overview of the various stages of growth and development of children and youth from a range of countries and all continents. The central theme of nutrition and physical fitness has been considered on the basis of the impact of negative and/or positive energy balance. Numerous points of view have been advanced, based on results gained through the utilization of a variety of accepted methodologies.

Numerous chapters addressed the growing concern for the increased prevalence of overweight and obesity amongst children and youth of many industrially developed countries. This is a major challenge for many countries including the relatively underdeveloped ones. Preservation of traditional practices in both nutrition and physical activity are generally the best guidelines to follow for the encouragement of optimal growth and development and maintenance of a desirable body composition. Unfortunately, an increasing number of societies for whom the modern western diet was unavailable in the past are now subjected to the very worst attributes of this diet, a preponderance of food low in nutritional value (but supposedly attractive and trendy for young people) and a less active life-style. Whilst a logical suggestion may appear to be reducing the recommended dietary allowance for children and youth, others believe that such an approach may not be ideal. Reinforcement of the latter position is provided in the knowledge that during the formative years, the level of spontaneous physical activity for the average child is higher than during other periods of life. Preservation of the spontaneity of movement in young children should be a key goal for all individuals. In situations where the self-regulation of dietary intake and physical activity on the part of children and youth has been reduced there is usually an enhanced prevalence of obesity and diabetes and also an increased exposure to risk factors for cardiovascular disease. In such situations, active interventions are imperative in which habitual physical activity and increased exercise are targeted thereby encouraging positive health and fitness.

In the Third World, efforts should continue to be directed at the achievement of the genetic potential of a population. Less commonly studied than maximizing the genetic potential of a population in relation to body size has been the functional capacity and physical fitness. Adaptation to malnutrition reflected in a 'small, but healthy individual' may not be considered an optimal scenario yet is eminently more desirable than 'small, unfit and sick'. Similarly, in situations where it is clear that the conditions necessary for the promotion of optimal growth and development cannot be met, the attainment of an adequate level of functional capacity and fitness may be a more realistic and achievable goal.

In summary, future research should continue to address the relationships between diet, physical activity, fitness, health and the environment of children and youth. An understanding of the characteristics of the young provides an important window of opportunity for future adults in society. It is imperative that research extends earlier guidelines, for example those comprising the framework of the International Biological Programme (IBP) and more recent work such as presented in this volume. In this way a concerted approach to the availability and understanding of various criteria and methods for widespread utilization can be maximized. There are so many questions to be resolved that continued scientific research of the pediatric years will continue to be dependent upon both interest and funding. Answers to a proportion of these questions could make a great contribution to the well-being of future generations all round the world.

Andrew Hills
Jana Pařízková

Subject Index

Age, effect on physical fitness variables 34–36, 39, 40, 54
Altitude, effects on physical performance
  aerobic performance 83–85
  anaerobic performance
    blood lactate concentration 88, 89
    force-velocity test 86
    oxygen debt 88
    Wingate test 86, 87
  growth effects 91
  nutritional status effects 79, 81, 82, 85, 86, 89–92
  socioeconomic status effects 80, 81, 85, 89
Anthropometry
  assessment methodology 158, 159
  Brazilian children 4, 6–9, 11
  Estonian children 70–72, 74
  Indian children 134
  Mozambique children 94, 95, 97, 98
  Senegalese children 118–121, 128, 130
  sex difference 56, 57
Arm circumference, correlating factors 29, 30
Australia
  body
    composition effects on weight control practices 50, 51
    image 47–50
  cardiovascular health 44, 45
  obesity in children 45–47

Balance, *see* Flamingo balance
Belgium, sex differences in physical performance 54–58, 61–65
Body image
  Australian children 47–50
  preschoolers in Brazil 4, 5, 11
  sex differences 47–50
Body mass index
  American vs Mexican children 13–16, 19, 20, 22–25
  components 14
  correlations with physical performance 19, 20, 22, 24, 25, 27
  measurement 15
  overweight
    classification analysis 20, 23
    comparison by ethnic group 17, 19, 23, 24
    definition 15, 23, 45, 46
  physical performance correlation in Senegalese children 123, 125, 128, 130
  radiation effects on children 106–108, 115
  statistical analysis 15, 16, 20, 22
  underweight
    classification analysis 20, 23
    comparison by ethnic group 17, 19, 23, 24
    definition 15, 23
Bolivia, altitude effects on physical performance
  aerobic performance 83–85

Bolivia, altitude effects on physical performance (continued)
  anaerobic performance
    blood lactate concentration 88, 89
    force-velocity test 86
    oxygen debt 88
    Wingate test 86, 87
  growth effects 91
  nutritional status
    evaluation 81, 82
    malnutrition effects 79, 85, 86, 89–92
  socioeconomic status effects 80, 81, 85, 89
Brazil
  anthropometric and performance characteristics of children 4, 6–9, 11
  body size, correlation with performance 4, 5, 9
  physical activity, children 3, 4, 8
  preschoolers
    body image 4, 5, 11
    motor perception 4, 5, 11
    nutrition 3–5, 8, 11
  public school physical education 2, 10
  skinfold thickness measurement 7, 8
  stature correlation with physical performance 9, 10
  survey
    food habits 2, 3
    socioeconomic background 2, 3
  zero order correlations among performance and psychological tests 5, 10

Cardiovascular disease, Australia 44, 45
Chernobyl
  cesium-137 half-life in adults and children 106
  radiation effects on children
    endurance 111, 114
    force abilities 110, 111, 114
    general health effects 108, 109, 115
    growth rate 107, 108, 115
    height 106–108
    physical work capacity index 109
    running abilities 110, 113, 114
    spirometry index 109
    throwing accuracy 111–113, 116
    weight 106–108
  radiation exposure levels 105
Chest circumference, correlating factors 30
Czech Republic, obesity prevention and treatment
  food reduction vs exercise 145, 150
  functional capacity of obese children 145–147
  summer treatment camp
    body composition outcomes 147–150, 153
    long-term effects 148, 149, 152, 153
    physical performance outcomes 147, 148, 150, 151

Diet, restriction in obesity treatment 145, 150, 161

Efficacy, assessment methods for children 156
Endurance, radiation effects on children 111, 114
Estonia
  anthropometric parameters of kindergarten children 70–72, 74
  physical activities of children 70, 72, 74
  physical activity, motor ability and anthropometric variable relationships 68–72, 74–77
  sex differences in physical performance 70, 72, 76, 77
Ethnic group
  effect on physical fitness variables 34–36
  effect on stature 29, 136, 137
EUROFIT test battery 54–56, 69

Flamingo balance, sex differences 57, 77
Force abilities, radiation effects on children 110, 111, 114

Grip strength
  correlating factors 30, 31, 36, 37, 39, 42, 76
  sex differences 56–58, 64, 76

Height, *see* Stature

India
  anthropometric measurements of children 134
  body composition and physical activity 132, 133, 137
  fitness evaluation of children
    aerobic capacity 132, 133, 135–139
    anaerobic capacity 141, 142
    maximum heart rate 136, 140
    oxygen pulse 140, 141
    ventilation in trained vs untrained children 136, 139
  height, comparison of children with other countries 136, 137
  weight, trained vs untrained children 136
International Biological Programme guidelines 162

Jumping performance, correlating factors 31, 32, 36, 37, 39

Menarche, age of onset 38, 127
Methodology, nutritional and physical assessment of children
  efficacy 156
  literature search 157–159
  outline of key issues and related questions 156
  reliability 156
  validity 156
Mexico
  body mass index comparisons with American children 13–16, 19, 20, 22–25
  physical performance comparison with Polish children 27–40, 42
Mozambique
  anthropometric measurements of children 94, 95, 97, 98
  nutritional status classification 96, 100–102
  physical activity correlation with nutrition 98–100
  physical fitness assessment 95, 96
  sex differences in physical performance 99–102

Obesity
  classification analysis 20, 23
  comparison by ethnic group 17, 19, 23, 24
  definition 15, 23, 45, 46
  food reduction vs exercise in treatment 145, 150, 161
  prevention in Australia 47
  summer treatment camp
    body composition outcomes 147–150, 153
    long-term effects 148, 149, 152, 153
    physical performance outcomes 147, 148, 150, 151
Overweight, *see* Body mass index, Obesity, Weight control

Percentage of variance, physical performance tests 33, 34, 39
Physical work capacity index, radiation effects on children 109
Poland, physical performance comparison with Mexican children 27–40, 42
Protein energy malnutrition, effects in children 1

Radiation, effects on children
  endurance 111, 114
  force abilities 110, 111, 114
  general health effects 108, 109, 115
  growth rate 107, 108, 115
  height 106–108
  physical work capacity index 109
  running abilities 110, 113, 114
  spirometry index 109
  throwing accuracy 111–113, 116
  weight 106–108
Reaction time, correlating factors 39, 42
Reliability, assessment methods for children 156
Running abilities, radiation effects on children 110, 113, 114
Running performance
  correlating factors 31, 36, 37, 42
  sex differences 57, 61, 63, 65

Subject Index

Senegal
  anthropometric measurements of children 118–121, 128, 130
  body mass index and physical performance 123, 125, 128, 130
  cardiorespiratory fitness of children 119, 122, 123, 128
  delay of adolescence 126, 127
  malnutrition 117, 118
  motor task performance 119, 121, 122, 128
Sex differences, physical performance
  anthropometric measurements 56, 57
  body image 47–50
  Brazilian children 4, 11
  Flemish youth 54–58, 61–65
  growth patterns 63, 66
  Mexican vs Polish children 29–36
  Mozambique children 99–102
  psychological factors 65, 66
Shuttle run, see Running performance
Skinfold thickness
  measurement 7, 8
  sex differences 63, 74
Spine flexibility index, correlating factors 32, 38

Spirometry index, radiation effects on children 109
Stature
  correlation with physical performance 9, 10, 29
  ethnic group effects 29, 136, 137
  radiation effects on children 106–108, 115
  sex differences in growth 63, 66

Throwing accuracy 111–113, 116

Underweight, see Body mass index
United States, body mass index comparisons with Mexican children 13–16, 19, 20, 22–25

Validity, assessment methods for children 156

Weight control, see also Obesity
  Australia 47
  food reduction vs exercise in obesity treatment 145, 150, 161
  influence of body composition 50, 51
Wingate test, altitude effects on anaerobic performance 86, 87

DATE DUE